SUCCESS STORIES

"When I started my waist was a size 42, today I'm a size 36. I lost 45 excess pounds. I don't use medication anymore for high blood pressure. It's a success."

R. Torres
Miami, FL

"My diabetes improved so much that I don't have to use insulin anymore, and I only use one medication to control my condition. Doing this helped me to recover my health, my metabolism, and my self-confidence. When I was overweight I wore a size 18 and today I'm a size 10."

M. Santiago
Chester, NY

"I had failed in so many different weight loss diets and systems that my husband told me that it wasn't worth it to keep on trying. Today I can wear size 6 clothes that I like, and I already gave away all of my size 14 clothes that I had in my closet. I will never go back to making the same mistakes as before."

T. Andreu
Carolina, PR

"My metabolism really improved. It was something that seemed impossible to me. Before my waist was a size 46 and now I buy size 36 pants."

P. Thomas
Camden, TX

"I was a horrible size 20. My children and friends criticized me. Everyone thought that my problem was that I ate a lot, but I learned that my problem was that I had a slow metabolism and a thyroid

condition that my doctors hadn't detected because it didn't show up in my lab tests. Learning about my metabolism allowed me to get the medical help that I needed. In getting that help and improving my habits and lifestyle, I successfully got down to my present size 8."

S. Rodríguez
Los Angeles, CA

"Frankly, I had already given up because no diet ever worked for me. I had done diets that count calories and had gone hungry. I didn't know that my problem was a slow metabolism. I have already lost almost 60 pounds and now my husband acts jealous because I look good again and men notice me. I was a size 16 and today I bought size 6 clothes that fit me beautifully."

M. Flores
San Juan, PR

"After I got married I gained about 30 pounds until I was a size 12. But the saddest part was that I started suffering from migraines, sinusitis, and even high blood pressure. My health deteriorated, and I always felt tired. Now I've gone back to wearing the clothes I wore when I first got married, size 6, and I have tons of energy. I recovered my metabolism."

Z. Adams
Charlotte, NC

"When I quit smoking, I gained almost 30 pounds. The cravings were killing me and I was eating sweets uncontrollably. With what I learned I successfully lost the same 30 pounds and I am at my normal size again. I did it without going hungry. It's a success."

M. Martínez
Guaynabo, PR

"I was addicted to sweets and carbohydrates, as well as to Coca-Cola. With what I learned I was able to break the bad habits, and

now I don't feel the need for the foods that made me so fat. I went from a size 16 down to my present size 8. I feel much more energetic and my migraines went away."

M. McCormick
Allentown, NJ

"I've been a diabetic for 12 years. With diabetes I gained weight and went from a size 4 up to a size 12. I felt sick and ugly. After doing this program I've successfully controlled my diabetes and I'm buying size 6 clothing. I still have a while left until I can get back to my original size 4, but I know I'm going to do it. This works!"

K. Sotomayor
San Juan, PR

"Finally, someone could explain to me the reasons for my slow metabolism. The most important thing is that I succeeded in improving my metabolism and I lost 36 pounds and 8 dress sizes in the process without going hungry or having cravings."

D. Angulo
Las Piedras, PR

The Power
Of Your
Metabolism

Warning:
This book, *The Power of Your Metabolism*, has been written only as a source of information. You should never consider the information found in this book as a substitute for the recommendations of your health professional or qualified physician. You should always talk to your doctor before beginning any diet, exercise, or health program. The author, Frank Suárez, is someone who has successfully overcome his own obesity; he is not a doctor, dietitian, or a nutritionist. He is a specialist in obesity and metabolism by his own merit. The information that this book provides is based upon the recommendations that throughout the last 20 years have been successful for the people that have sought out his help in losing weight and recovering their metabolism. We have made reasonable efforts so that all of the information described here is truthful. The majority of the information is based on the experiences acquired through working with thousands of people in the NaturalSlim system.

This book is dedicated to my loving wife, Elizabeth, who is also my best friend and ally.

I also dedicate this book to my favorite philosopher, educator, and researcher, L. Ron Hubbard, who served as an inspiration and as an example of the ability to observe life, as well as the importance of the unending search for truth.

CONTENTS

INTRODUCTION

After 20 years of practicing medicine, I have seen how patients have suffered the consequences of obesity. There are multiple complications that being overweight can bring: arthritis, depression, heart complications, hypertension, problems with the liver, diabetes, etc. and the list goes on. For many years I saw how patients carried on with different diets that did not work or that, after a short while of having produced some result, the weight would come back and sometimes even more than what was lost. I witnessed their desperation and how their problem affected them day after day. They believed their lives to be ruined because they had no energy and were suffering with the complications that come with obesity.

There are an enormous variety of diets designed to lose weight, but many patients found these to be difficult to follow for extended periods of time without ending up exhausted by them. They would begin with enthusiasm, but surely lost motivation along the way. Some diets were better than others and were designed with the best of intentions, but because they were complicated or grueling, patients could not lose weight or keep it off.

I thought the ideal diet would consist of a simple method that would be easy to follow, where you could eat everything, and thus my patients would be able to follow it for the rest of their lives without falling into apathy. In other words, a change in their nutrition or better said, an improvement in their "lifestyle". I studied many methods of weight loss with special interest in the Mediterranean diet. These countries have the lowest percentages of obesity and heart disease in the world. What my patients really needed to do was find a diet that worked.

Several of my patients who suffered from obesity, amongst these diabetics, had managed to lose weight while reducing the need for prescribed medication with the help of the NaturalSlim system. I was curious and began to look into the subject and found that what they were learning regarding the metabolism and nutrition was logical and was producing improvements in health, plus it was adapting perfectly to the necessities of my patients. I then realized that the book *The Power of Your Metabolism* explained, in a sample way the common-sense concepts that were being used in NaturalSlim. I began to recommend this type of diet and it simply worked. My patients found it easy to follow and were losing weight. The doses of medication were being reduced and more importantly, they were eating all kinds of food and it made it possible to continue on the diet indefinitely. It is immensely gratifying to see how a patient makes changes to improve his life and see how hope comes back. It filled me with happiness to see how they understood that they could take control of their body again and that they would not end up a pile of illnesses and complaints.

This book presents a simple, practical and easy method of nutrition that is easy to follow and more importantly, is that from what I have seen, it works for anybody. It is a new point of view, but it is all encompassing and does not limit itself to strictly "diets" but is based on combining different factors that improve the metabolism and health of the human body. This book has a strong dose of "common sense" that will positively affect our patients who are overweight, obese or diabetic. A medical doctor's goal is the physical and mental well-being of his patients. The happiness and enthusiasm that is brought by observing these patients improve their health has no comparison.

I congratulate Mr. Frank Suárez for taking health and well-being to so many patients who are in need of it.

Carlos M. Cidre, MD
Internal Medicine Specialist
Board Certified

A HUGE PROBLEM

Important Note

The purpose of this book is to help educate you on the subject of the metabolism. Whether you are trying to lose weight or improve your health, having and understanding the correct information is vital.

For this reason, should you have any questions along the way, please do not hesitate to call or email us using the contact information below. We have a team of Certified Metabolism Consultants that are ready to answer any questions or uncertainties you may have! This a free service offered to help you achieve your goals.

We also offer a free metabolism evaluation to help you begin your weight loss or health journey. Simply call or email us using the below information to get started.

We look forward to hearing from you!

Sincerely,
The NaturalSlim Team

CONTACT INFO

Phone: 888-348-7352
Email: Info@relaxslim.com
Website: www.us.NaturalSlim.com

Author's Notes

My goal is to put out a message that serves to increase or restore your energy, your metabolism, and your health in general. The written message is communicated through words. The words have meanings that aren't always known by all of us.

This is why I did everything I could to avoid technical words or medical terms in this book. Whenever I find myself forced to use a technical word I make sure to provide the definition for it so that the reader doesn't lose interest in the subject and so that they can understand it. In reality "knowledge is power", but the knowledge is acquired through the words of the language used.

When I find myself obligated to use a word that I think could be misunderstood, I have included its definition in the bottom of the page where I first use it. There are also other word definitions that are in the section: GLOSSARY—DEFINITIONS OF WORDS towards the end of the book. The idea is that you can find any words that are new to you in the bottom of the page or in the glossary without having to use a medical or specialized dictionary. Nevertheless, it is always a good idea to have a decent dictionary available, because, even a common word of our language, that you don't understand, can make you lose interest in what you are reading.

If at any point during the reading of this book you find yourself becoming sleepy, groggy or suddenly feeling tired, just look for the word or words that you don't understand in what you just read and clarify their meaning in the glossary or dictionary. Words convey specific meanings that help us achieve knowledge. But, when words are misunderstood they represent a barrier to acquiring knowledge. Thus, understanding the correct meaning and use of the words is the key to our understanding of any subject.

It Was A Personal Problem

I've had problems with my weight since a very young age. I was always "chunky". In high school I went to an all-boys military school where my classmates made fun of me because of my weight. They had a nickname for me that wasn't very nice (printing the word is not allowed), that had to do with a part of my body.

Because I was "chunky", slow, and uncoordinated, I didn't participate in any sports at my school. I got used to the idea of being a spectator.

The social life I remember from this time was full of rejection, including the rejection from the girls that danced with me just because I was a good dancer, even though I was "fat". Beyond getting them to dance with me, it was difficult to initiate a relationship. One way or another I felt like I was trapped in being fat and over the years I learned to accept it as something that was inevitable.

Luckily, I was talented in music. I learned to play the saxophone and succeeded in getting the attention of some girls. Over time, I started a relationship, got married, had 4 children, and continued my professional life, but always feeling fatter than usual.

Some 25 years after I left college and began to work, I had kept on gaining weight little by little. Not only was I 40 pounds overweight, but also, my doctor, a personal friend of mine, warned me that my blood pressure, cholesterol, and triglycerides[1] were out of control. He also warned me that I was at the point of developing diabetes.

---

[1] Triglycerides – They are fats. Blood fats are called triglycerides. See the glossary for a more complete definition.

Such severe warnings from my friend and doctor made me react and I decided to do something about it; little did I know what awaited me.

I sought out professional help. I went on a diet of limiting calories and I lost 20 pounds, but I felt hungry all the time because this diet was one of those in which I was always eating less than my body craved. Willpower was a vital element in bringing it to an end. Even though I had lost 20 pounds and only had 20 more to go to reach my goal, I eventually stopped following the diet because I had stalled at a certain weight plateau. Even though I was following the diet, I simply couldn't lose any more weight. I was discouraged and stopped following it. In the next 3 months I gained back the 20 pounds that I had lost and an additional 10 or 12 more. In other words, I had rebounded back and forth like a yo-yo.

Some months later I decided to try a vegetarian diet and became a vegan. I lost weight, but again I got to the point where the weight loss was stagnant, and I felt weak. Again, I was discouraged, and I stopped the diet. In a short amount of time I went back to gaining the lost weight, and then some.

Sometime after I made other attempts, including jogging, which made me lose a lot of weight, until one day I injured myself while running and had to give it up. The lost weight came back quite rapidly.

My attempts in losing weight had turned into a constant torture. Even so, I kept on trying other diets and systems. One of the diets that I tried was the famous Atkins diet, a diet where you only eat meat and fat. On this diet I lost a lot of weight, 35 pounds, but one day I passed out and woke up in the emergency room. After that scare, something told me that a diet of just meat and fat couldn't be healthy for me.

After the scare with the Atkins diet I decided that I had to have a better understanding of my metabolism. My desire to lose weight had turned almost into an obsession and I wasn't ready to give up. I gave myself the task of studying the subject of the metabolism and everything related to nutrition, digestion, and any other topic that in some way could help me understand and solve my problem with obesity. The study of the subject of obesity became my hobby and my only topic of interest outside of my family and work.

I remember spending at least 8 years reading and researching EVERYTHING that I could find about diets, obesity, metabolism, the biology of the body, cells, digestion, and a thousand other related subjects. I spent many hours on the Internet. I bought hundreds of books about dieting, nutrition, and the metabolism. I explored the medical aspects of obesity to see if there was some sickness that caused it. I studied many subjects, including some not normally considered related to obesity, in my search for clues to this problem.

The search for the causes and solutions to obesity became the main focus of my life. The subjects of obesity and metabolism were a true challenge for me. Each day after completing my work in my sales job, I devoted myself to what became my other job, reading and studying about obesity and metabolism. I took notes, I made files by subject, and I wrote my thoughts and conclusions. I did experiments with my body taking different supplements and natural herbs to see if I could find the ones that would make me "thin".

Little by little and almost without realizing it, I was losing weight. I lost the extra 40 pounds that I had put on. At this point my lab tests came back normal. My blood pressure was normal, as well as my triglycerides and cholesterol. Besides losing weight and getting my health back, I realized that acquiring the knowledge about so many subjects related to obesity had changed me. I started to see that "everything is connected with everything" in the human body. I learned that obesity couldn't be overcome from just the limited perspective of food. Fasting or eating less doesn't necessarily solve the problem of obesity. I found that there are multiple factors that decrease the metabolism and cause obesity. It's not just the food factor, like a nutritionist might think. I discovered the METABOLISM.

My friends and acquaintances saw that I had lost a lot of weight and many of them were interested in asking me what I did to lose the weight. It occurred to me that I should write up a summary of my discoveries and every time someone asked me how I did it, I'd simply hand them the 7 pages of written summary so that they could try it. I thought that giving them the written summary with my recommendations for losing weight would solve the problem of having to explain everything that I had discovered. I was wrong. The written summary worked for them, but it also opened up numerous other doubts with respect to their own weight loss, and they always ended up calling me to set up an appointment for a "personal consultation". Perhaps this happened because the subjects of dieting and metabolism contain the most failures and disillusions in the world. The majority of people have failed in various attempts to lose weight. Therefore, they feel hopeful when they read something that offers them the opportunity to eliminate the thousand and one contradictions that they have read and heard about the subject, as well as the memories of their own failures in losing weight.

The field of obesity and metabolism is a controversial one; there are millions of different experts with certifications, diplomas, and qualifications, and that, oddly enough, contradict each other with total neglect. My personal observation is that the general public ends up in a state of confusion of having so many expert opinions that contradict each other. Some "experts" talk about calories while others say that obesity is a sickness and try to treat it with medications. Some claim that the only thing that works is physical exercise and others, that don't have solutions, blame the entire problem of obesity on hereditary factors. Overall, clear solutions didn't exist.

By this time, the number of people that called me to ask for my help kept on growing, since some of them had taken up the habit of making copies of my written recommendations and passing them along to their friends and family. Each day more people called me, people even called me from far away towns because somehow, they had gotten a copy of my recommendations. Many of these individuals were already in a state of despair because they had tried everything and hadn't found a solution to their obesity problem. Various people, especially women, were already affected emotionally by the constant failure of their diets, and the accusations and criticisms from those who, not understanding the subject of metabolism, accused them of overeating.

The constant calls and "personal consultations" made me realize that I had hit a real ruin. Obesity is an emotional topic full of failures, confusion, and incomplete information. I decided to create a company in order to dedicate myself to helping these people overcome their obesity. It was sort of crazy because I wasn't a nutritionist or a doctor. I only had my knowledge and the successful results of those whom I'd consulted. I accepted it as a new challenge and created NaturalSlim (www.us.NaturalSlim.com). I called it NaturalSlim, "The weight lost that stays lost", because my intention was to change the knowledge and lifestyle of the members of the system. Experience has shown me that the only thing that lasts forever is KNOWLEDGE. I decided that NaturalSlim would be a knowledge center where thousands of people could educate themselves on the subject of obesity and metabolism. I bet that the knowledge would be of more value and more use in the long term than any supplement or frozen food. I also bet that the knowledge of the causes of obesity and its solutions would provoke a change in people, because, in knowing about these subjects, their conscience would get to them if they didn't do it right. It was a real risk, but it turned out well; NaturalSlim became a success because it produces what is most desired: RESULTS.

In my own case, I had attained results that weren't only reflected in my weight and my waistline. They were results that demonstrated a significant improvement in my health. I had given up being "fat", tired, and weak to turn myself into someone thin and full of enthusiasm. I had recovered my metabolism and my health.

BEFORE	AFTER
CHOLESTEROL 290 (high level)	CHOLESTEROL 140 (Normal)
TRIGLYCERIDES 345 (very high)	TRIGLYCERIDES 90 (Normal)
BLOOD PRESSURE 140/100 (High)	BLOOD PRESSURE 120/80 (Normal)
WEIGHT 207 Pounds	WEIGHT 166 Pounds
WAIST SIZE: 41	WAIST SIZE: 35

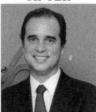

Some friends recommend that I not give out all of the information to the members of the NaturalSlim system because if I did then they wouldn't need us anymore. It's logical to think that one who has learned their lessons in college will eventually stop needing to go to the classes. I resisted this idea to restrict the education of our members because I thought that the things that had been discovered, in reality, produced such amazing results that the same members of the system would recommend us to their family members and friends. Looking at the national statistics on obesity, which each year are rising, I realized that I wouldn't be left without potential clients for a long time. I decided to give each member of NaturalSlim a complete education about the metabolism, trusting in that, as they applied it, the positive results would attract other people who also wanted to lose weight and recover their metabolism. By luck, that is how it went. NaturalSlim has more than hundreds of thousands of members and keeps on growing. It's true: happy clients are the best advertising!

Now, NaturalSlim is a complete system where the technology to recover the metabolism and energy of the body has been developed to an optimum point and it is almost impossible for a person to not be able to lose weight on the NaturalSlim system. Today, dozens of doctors refer their patients to NaturalSlim when they want them to lose weight in a natural way. Many of the doctors that recommend us have been members of the NaturalSlim system and came to us motivated by the results that they saw in their patients.

I have to say that I don't think any other job exists that provides as much satisfaction as my job as Executive Director of NaturalSlim. I constantly have the opportunity to see how the members of the NaturalSlim system lose weight and improve their health so much that, in many cases they don't need to use medications anymore. Nearly every week we see diabetics that don't need to use insulin anymore and people who were very sick and weak that, today, have recovered their health entirely. My job at NaturalSlim is one that is very gratifying and full of satisfaction in being able to help others.

This book, *The Power of Your Metabolism*, is oriented toward all of those people that want to take control of their weight in a natural and healthy way. If you want to reduce your clothing size, this book will definitely help you. If you want to maintain your weight, here you will find the facts that will allow you to do so. But, in honor of the truth, I must say that for those of you who have experienced great difficulties in losing weight, it is possible that you require intensive and personalized help. NaturalSlim specializes in offering help to the "difficult cases". For example, in NaturalSlim there are natural treatments against yeasts and parasites that you can't provide in a book, and we have seen that some people can't lose weight because their bodies are severely infected by parasitic organisms. NaturalSlim offers natural hormonal help for those women whose irregular menstruation reflects their hormonal disorders. In some cases, people don't lose weight because they have digestive problems, and this is another area in which NaturalSlim offers help. In addition, NaturalSlim provides a follow up and personal motivation that ends up being vital for those people whose multiple failures have lowered their self-esteem and perseverance. When people have failed numerous times in trying to lose weight, it makes them give up a lot easier in any new attempt because their hopes have been shattered so many times; it's human nature.

So, this book communicates some truths that produce noticeable benefits for those people that apply them. It doesn't guarantee results because it wouldn't be honest to guarantee results. There are people who have health conditions that cause difficulties in losing weight. What is guaranteed is that these truths have been applied by more than hundreds of thousands of people with excellent results, and at times, exceptional results for the majority.

These topics, obesity and metabolism were a "personal problem" that I had; now they are my life and they fill me with the enormous satisfaction of having helped thousands of people to be free of the fat trap called "obesity". There definitely isn't anything more satisfying than helping others.

WEIGHT PROBLEMS AND OBESITY: EPIDEMICS

Weight problems and obesity have grown to epidemic proportions, or at least this is how the United States Department of Health has publicly described it.

It is calculated that 68.0% of the population is overweight and that 24.7% (1 in every 4 people) are already obese. The term "obesity" doesn't mean the same thing as "being overweight". "Obesity" means that you are at least 20% over the normal weight for your height. All obese people are overweight, but not all people who are overweight are obese.

What is certain is that these statistics about the population are getting worse. For example, look at this graph:

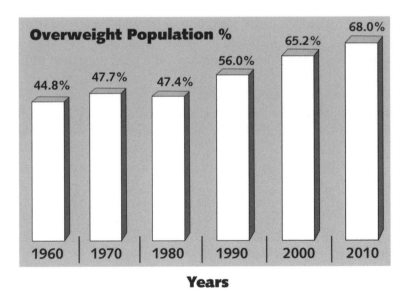

Source: National Health and Nutrition Examination Survey Data. Hyattsville, MD.

In fact, childhood obesity has been constantly rising for many decades and the same has happened with juvenile diabetes. It has been shown that a direct relationship exists between being overweight and having diabetes. It is calculated that more than 85% of diabetics are overweight. Any diabetic that manages to lose weight experiences a substantial improvement in their diabetic condition.

The American Cancer Society has published studies that show much higher incidence of cancer amongst people who are overweight. To mention some examples, overweight women experience 112% higher incidence of breast cancer. Overweight men experience 352% higher incidence of liver cancer (Source: NAASO, *The Obesity Society, Study on Obesity*). In other words, being overweight is a true risk to your health.

In conclusion, we can say without a doubt that we are losing the battle against obesity at a national level. Each day there are more obese people. Because obesity is related to high blood pressure, high triglycerides, high cholesterol, and diabetes, statistics also reflect annual increases in these conditions. The sales of medications to treat these conditions are a good indication of the magnitude of the problem. In the last 10 years, pharmaceutical companies have broken their own record of sales of medications associated with these conditions. It's a shame to say it, but the obese and sick are good business for the pharmaceutical companies.

All of this is happening while our stores are stocking up on foods that are "sugar free", "fat free", "low fat", and "low calorie". An interesting bit of information is that federal government studies, like the NHANES, show that we currently consume about 19% less fat than 40 years ago; however, we are now 47% more overweight than in that era.

When you understand the way in which the body creates fat you will realize that our population isn't more overweight than before as a result of us eating more fat than before. There are other reasons why the proportion of fat is increasing in our bodies, which will be discussed in the section of "How fat is created in the body". This is information that everyone who wants to avoid being overweight or obese should know.

Lastly, we must see that the future of our youth is increasingly more uncertain due to the epidemic of weight problems and obesity. There are already hundreds of thousands of boys and girls that need to use prescription medications to control high blood pressure and cholesterol. We are creating a new generation of weak, overweight, flaccid bodies that only have enough energy to play with electronic games. We are setting a very bad example of what they should learn about nutrition and the proper caring of their bodies. Even the food served in school cafeterias is appalling, with pizza, hot dogs, and other things that could be called "non-food".

It is said that obesity has a certain hereditary factor. I agree, to a certain extent. I agree that there is a strong hereditary factor, but this factor has <u>nothing to do with our genes or chromosomes</u>. It does have to do with the fact that children inherit the bad habits of their parents. A family with bad habits raises children with bad habits. All of the hundreds of overweight children, which I have worked with, lived in homes where unhealthy nutrition and unhealthy lifestyles were the obvious causes of the child's obesity.

It is evident that none of us has the power to change all of society. Nevertheless, each one of us does have the power to increase our knowledge and the level of responsibility as to what we feed our loved ones. If everyone takes responsibility themselves to improve their own immediate family, and the rest of the world does the same, in no time, we will have made the whole society better. What is certain is that if we don't do anything with respect to this problem, not even with our loved ones, we will have been accomplices to the creation of the deficient states of health of our loved ones and our future generations.

DIETS, THE KINGDOM OF CONTRADICTIONS

There are topics that are controversial by nature. Subjects like politics and religion. But the subject of diets, besides being controversial, is full of contradictions. The contradictions between different diets go from eating a lot of fat, a lot of protein[2], and almost no amount of carbohydrates (Atkins diet), to the recommendation of exactly the opposite, eating no fat, little or no protein, and tons of carbohydrates (Pritikin diet). As a result, the public is generally in a state of confusion on the topic of diets.

The reality is that when a person goes to a bookstore with the hope of finding a book on dieting, they find themselves completely confused because of the never-ending variety of diets that exist today. Every one of the books claims to have "the best diet" and many of the books are written by people with degrees in medicine, nutrition, physics, or chemistry. They all recommend some sort of diet that will solve everything for the person who wants to lose weight. There are approaches as varied as controlling calories, reducing fat consumption, vegetarianism, fruit juice diets, diets to eliminate dairy products or wheat, diets of consuming only organic or natural products, and a thousand others. In the end: confusion.

Then, there are the most well-known diets: "Atkins Diet", "Scarsdale Diet", "Pritikin Diet", "South Beach Diet", "Sugar Busters Diet", "Caveman Diet", and the list continues; it is never-ending. In my search to find which diet worked the best for me to lose weight, I think I tried practically all of them. I found that the diet that made me lose weight the best was that of Doctor Atkins, who has a diet

---

[2] Protein - proteins are foods like meat, cheese, and eggs. Proteins are made up of amino acids. Several amino acids together build a protein. Many hormones, like insulin, are proteins. Digestive enzymes are also proteins that are made up of amino acids. The word "protein" originates from the Greek word *"protas"*, which means "of utmost importance".

low in carbohydrates. But I noticed that this diet made me horribly weak. I even got sick. I finally came to the conclusion that it is an extreme diet and you can't use it as a "way of life" because it is too limited in the selection of foods and it uses too many red meats and bacon that aren't necessarily the best type of nutrients for the body.

Searching for alternatives, I was interested to find that the people from the Mediterranean Sea statistically have the least cases of obesity and heart problems. This got me thinking that I should see what type of food they eat in the Mediterranean[3]. I also observed that the Mediterranean Diet lets you eat everything without abusing refined carbohydrates like bread, rice and sugar. In the Mediterranean they eat a lot of fish and seafood, a lot of salad and hard textured kind of bread that is very rich in fiber. They drink wine, eat cheese every day, and use hams like "prosciutto", a type of sliced ham. In this area the people don't use huge quantities of sugar. In these countries they enjoy butter and practically everyone cooks with olive oil. I figured I could learn from them.

I was experimenting with different food proportions and found that if you reduce refined carbohydrates (bread, flour, rice, potatoes, grits, sweets, sugars, etc.) you can lose weight without needing to eliminate carbohydrates completely. I realized that it was really a question of the QUALITY of the carbohydrates than the quantity of them. I found that if I reduced the industrial oils, like corn and vegetable oil, and substituted them with olive oil, I could lose weight. Eating vegetables and salads also turned out to be of help. I found that a moderate diet with a reduction of refined carbohydrates, accompanied by good proteins (chicken, turkey, fish and seafood) and lots of water, produced a significant feeling of well-being.

---

[3] The Mediterranean refers to the area where the Mediterranean Sea is located, where the countries of Italy, Greece, Israel, and Egypt can be found.

Afterwards, when I created NaturalSlim, I applied this knowledge and began to see impressive results in people that were eating this way. Person after person was losing their fat and they always had more energy without experiencing hunger or cravings.

So, the basic concept of a Mediterranean Diet was what worked for thousands and thousands of people. Good proteins (meat, fish, seafood, whey protein), vegetables, salads, cheese, eggs, and a minimum of bread, flour, rice, starches (potato, sweet potato, tapioca, etc.) and very little sugar. I discovered that we didn't have to have any "prohibitions". It is a matter of reducing those foods that decrease the metabolism and, additionally, makes us fat: refined carbohydrates.

WHAT IS YOUR METABOLISM, REALLY?

A number of people complain about having a "slow metabolism", but what actually is the metabolism?

The definitions in the dictionary for the word metabolism can be too technical or complex. I offer my readers the following basic definition of "metabolism" that I find easier to understand:

Metabolism: all the movements, changes and actions that your body does to convert food and nutrients into energy in order to survive.

There are many processes, movements, actions and changes that the human body carries out to be able to survive: digestion, absorption, breathing, immune system (defense), circulation, elimination, etc. Each one of these processes has something in common: *movement*. The movement always involves the use of energy. Without energy there isn't movement. All matter is made of energy in *movement*. Although we can't see the atoms that make up the matter moving in their constant orbits, it is still true that all of matter is made up of atoms that are in *movement*.

The human body is made up of matter. There are components like water, fat, proteins, carbohydrates and minerals. All of these matters are animated by the life in us, but, at the same time, they respond to the laws of physics and atoms. In order to survive, all live organisms must be able to have *movement*, but the *movement* must be an ordered *movement* and at the right rate. For example, if our heart beats at a rate that is too slow, it would be a risk almost as severe as if it were beating at a rate that is too fast. In order to survive, the human body needs to have *movement,* but this movement must be at an adequate rate, not too slow, not too fast.

The metabolism is a sum of all the *movements* that the body executes to be able to exist as a body. When we say that we have a "slow metabolism", in reality we are saying that the *movement* of the body isn't at the optimal *rate.*

There is health, nutrition, and lifestyle factors that reduce the *rate* of the *movement* of the body's processes. Other factors also exist that accelerate and contribute to increasing the *rate* of the *movement* of the body's processes.

People associate the so-called: "slow metabolism" with a severe difficulty in losing weight. However, having a "slow metabolism" is something that can become quite dangerous. This is because when the metabolism is too slow all the processes of the body are also slowed and that can cause constipation, accumulation of toxins, bad circulation, lots of infections, bad digestion, weight problems, and obesity, among other things.

The Power of Your Metabolism is about how to recognize these factors and how to utilize the knowledge about them with respect to improving your metabolism, and with it, your health.

THE EVER SO FAMOUS SLOW METABOLISM

The statistics don't lie. The great majority of the population is overweight and one in every four people is already obese. The biggest problem is that the trend is clear: the situation keeps worsening year after year.

It is calculated that at any time of the year, more than 30% of the population is doing some type of diet, exercise program or effort to lower or control their weight. However, we are losing the battle; the statistics show that the population keeps getting fatter with every year that goes by. Since weight problems and obesity bring about other health problems like high blood pressure, high cholesterol and diabetes, these health conditions are also increasing as well.

Many people that have tried several of the many different popular diets have already given up because they observed that they made the effort but saw very poor results. Others get depressed when they see how a family member or friend who is thin eats everything that they themselves can't eat and yet continues being thin, even though they eat candy, chocolate, and ice cream every day.

It is something illogical because for some mysterious reason it seems like some of us get fat "just from looking at food". This phenomenon is called the "slow metabolism". The term "slow metabolism" has gotten popular at such a level that just about any person that sees that he or she gains weight easily or that has great difficulty in losing weight uses it to describe their condition even though they might not be able to explain what the word "metabolism" means. For the population "slow metabolism" means eat a little and gain a lot.

If we look at the national statistics of weight problems and obesity we have to conclude that it is obvious that the number of people that experience the infamous "slow metabolism" is rising. Now the only thing left to understand is which factors are those that decrease our metabolism and turn it into a "slow metabolism". Then we could not only avoid a "slow metabolism", but also recover our metabolism and bring it to an optimal point of health and energy.

This reminds me of not too long ago when I spoke with a very pretty young woman that was holding a beautiful baby in her arms. She told me about her great difficulty in losing weight. She explained to me that before having her baby she could eat anything and always maintained her figure. She showed me photos of a time when she used to wear a slender size 4 and with tears in her eyes she told me "now I'm a size 10 and nothing looks good on me". Her anguish was obvious. Then she said, "I have a slow metabolism". I also remember a diabetic man who was at least 60 pounds overweight who told me "I was one of those skinny people who ate like a horse and never got fat." This formerly skinny guy who is now severely overweight complained of having a "slow metabolism".

What are the factors that decrease the metabolism and turn it into a slow metabolism? We'll find out further on in the book. The most important thing is to notice the solutions. In other words, what we can do to recover the most out of our metabolism.

After having worked with more than hundreds of thousands of people to help them recover their metabolism, I can tell you in advance that there are various factors that lower your metabolism. The agile metabolism that almost all of us are born with can suffer damage if we don't take care of it. Once it has suffered damage it could then become what we call a "slow metabolism". Not all of the damage to the metabolism is recoverable, but a good part of it is. In other words, if we can't recover 100% of the metabolism from when we were younger, we can recover a substantial part by applying the right knowledge. So, there is hope for everyone of any age. I've seen a 72-year-old woman apply the right guidelines to increase her metabolism and she successfully went from an enormous size 22 to an elegant size 10. Her family couldn't believe it; the woman, who before could only walk with the help of a cane, today walks 1 mile 3 times a week without any help, while being full of energy and enthusiasm.

Of course, there are various "experts" who insist on the fixed and wrong idea that the only reason that people are overweight or obese is because they consume too many calories. Generally, they stick to the simplistic idea that nutrition is the only aspect that must be improved in order to successfully lose weight and feel good. There are people who certainly can have good intentions, but surely don't have the capacity of observing the multiple factors that affect the metabolism of a person. At times the need of some of our health professionals "to be correct" overpowers their own curiosity and common sense. In my case, I was a victim of my own obesity and I couldn't have the luxury of closing myself off to this idea that just by going hungry and "counting calories" I could lose weight. My mental health and self-esteem were at play with this subject of the metabolism.

Most people only think of a diet when they want to lose weight. The idea that nutrition is the only or main area to improve when one wants to lose weight is a limited one. It is true that the diet you use is a very important factor indeed. But the diet has to do only with food and food could be called the body's fuel. In this sense food is to a body like gasoline is to your car. On the other hand, the metabolism, which is what converts food (the body's fuel) into energy, is more like your car's motor. Having a "slow metabolism" is like having problems with your car's motor that can't be solved solely by improving the fuel (diet). To solve the problem of a "slow metabolism", you have to understand the metabolism (the motor). This is why so many people fail in their diets; they don't understand how the metabolism works and thus ignore it.

Having a "slow metabolism" doesn't have to be a life-sentence. Your metabolism, for the most part, can be recovered if you stop doing the things that decrease it and start doing the things that increase it.

RELEVANT AND VITAL INFORMATION

It could be said that there is a large amount of information (knowledge, tips, techniques) that one should know in order to turn a "slow metabolism" into a faster one. This information can be classified in two types:

- Relevant information
- Vital information

In every subject there are degrees of importance. For example, in the subject of having a successful marriage you must both be faithful to your spouse and also be good with the little details like remembering anniversary dates. But, in terms of the importance of each characteristic it is much more "vital" to be faithful than to be good at remembering anniversary dates. Remembering the anniversary date could be called "relevant information" because it has some importance and being faithful would certainly be part of the "vital information" to having a successful marriage.

In this subject of the metabolism, the "relevant" information is the information about those things that have to do with your metabolism and with overcoming being overweight that have been proven useful in improving or protecting the metabolism. In other words, "relevant" information is information like: how moderate exercise is beneficial in losing weight, the advantages of consuming white meats (chicken, turkey, fish) instead of red meats (beef, pork), the kinds of water that will increase the metabolism (tap water, distilled, spring, filtered, etc.) and many others which are discussed. Within the subject of the metabolism there is a lot of relevant information that people should know and the intent of this book is to explain all of it. The relevant information is what we should know in order to help us increase the body's metabolism.

Now, the vital information is <u>very important information</u> and without it you will not be able to increase or recover your metabolism at all. The vital information is the most important information to know about this subject and it is knowledge that if applied correctly guarantees that you will be successful, and the lack of this knowledge guarantees your failure. It is vital!

Throughout this book I will identify for you which information is classified as "vital". The idea is to help you distinguish the relative importance between all of the factors that increase or decrease your metabolism. It's possible to succeed in increasing your metabolism even if you disregard some relevant information, but it is certain that you will fail in your attempt if you ignore any of the vital information. Therefore, I will identify each subject that is vital as vital information, so that you can assign it the importance that it should have.

If the subject isn't identified as vital information, you can consider it relevant information. If the subject of the chapter is vital information, it will be identified in this way at the beginning of the subject:

THIS IS VITAL INFORMATION

You can be successful in increasing your metabolism and losing weight even if you don't apply some of the relevant information. However, I guarantee you that you will fail in your efforts if you ignore any of the vital information. In other words, everything can seem important, but not all of it has the same magnitude of importance when it comes to achieving your goal of recovering your metabolism and losing weight. If you ignore the vital information you simply will not succeed.

Naturally, we each have a body that is different from everyone else. You have your own unique body that no one else has. There are different degrees of "slow metabolisms". There are metabolisms that are a little slow, there are those that are noticeably slow and those that are extremely slow, where the person practically feels like they gain weight "just from looking at food". Meanwhile, the slower a metabolism is, the more important it is to apply all of the relevant and vital information about the metabolism in order to succeed. People that have an extremely slow metabolism will have to be more disciplined in applying all of the possible help factors to successfully overcome being overweight or obese.

THE ENEMIES
OF YOUR
METABOLISM

FACTORS THAT DECREASE THE METABOLISM

People that fail in diets question what it is that they are doing wrong. Some people have such a "slow metabolism", that no amount of sacrifice gives them results.

Of course, the people that have a "slow metabolism" generally believe that the only thing that they should have to do to lose weight is to modify their diet. This has been the biggest mistake, thinking that the only thing that you have to do to lose weight is to modify what you eat.

Nutrition is an important factor, but it is also true that there are other factors that decrease the metabolism. This is why people that have a "slow metabolism" can't lose weight, even though they greatly reduce or vary their consumption of food. It is obvious that nutrition can't be the only factor that affects the metabolism when there are those famous thin people that can eat whatever they want (candies, chocolates, desserts, breads, greasy foods) and yet they never put on weight. If it were true that all obesity is a result of what you eat, then all of those thin people who can eat whatever they want would also be the fattest people in the world! The existence of these "skinny overeaters" contrasts with the sad reality of those other people that seem to "gain weight just from looking at food" because they have a "slow metabolism".

There are various factors that decrease the metabolism that if combined, can contribute to a person beginning to suffer from a "slow metabolism". It is of benefit to know about those factors that reduce our metabolism because knowing about them can help us avoid or conquer the infamous "slow metabolism". Having an agile or optimum metabolism is also a guarantee that you will be in good health.

EXCESS SUGAR AND REFINED CARBOHYDRATES

The epidemics of weight and obesity problems are caused by various factors that lower the metabolism. Perhaps the most evident of these factors is the excessive use of sugars and refined carbohydrates (bread, pasta, flour, rice, sweets, chocolates, candies, etc.).

I should clarify that carbohydrates are necessary foods. However, there are different qualities of carbohydrates: natural carbohydrates and refined carbohydrates. Natural carbohydrates are those that are in their natural state without having been industrially manipulated by humans. Examples are vegetables and fruits. Refined carbohydrates are modern products created by the food industry that have gone through a variety of polishing, bleaching, grinding and refining.

Within the natural carbohydrates there are some carbohydrates that have a very sweet flavor. The sweet carbohydrates can come from "natural" sources but the fact that they are sweet indicates that they are very high in sugars like *fructose* [4] that can turn into fat. Examples of very sweet carbohydrates can be fruits like bananas, mangoes, and raisins.

---

[4] Fructose - Fructose is a monosaccharide (simple sugar). Fructose can be found in most vegetables and fruits. It is processed in the liver. When too much fructose enters the liver, the liver can't process it all fast enough for the body to use as sugar. Instead, it starts making fats from the fructose and sending them off into the bloodstream as triglycerides.

There are fruits that aren't excessively sweet like strawberries, apples and pears, which are acceptable as "natural" carbohydrates.

When carbohydrates are industrially processed they lose a good part of their nutritional value (vitamins and minerals) and they turn into foods that can easily make us fat. For example, the most nutritious part of wheat is the germ, which is where the grain has all of its vitamins and minerals. The germ is extracted from the wheat during the industrial process, and what we end up consuming is only the starch (simple sugar) of the wheat. Manufacturers of vitamins buy wheat germ and extract from it part of the vitamins that they later sell us in their vitamin tablets and capsules.

The industrial processes to refine carbohydrates (wheat, rice, corn) are rather harsh. The food manufacturers have only one thing in mind: their profit. Carbohydrates that are already refined are turned into wheat flour, corn meal, corn syrup, instant mashed potatoes, soy flour and other forms of refined carbohydrates. These foods are so refined, and their molecules are so small that the human body quickly turns them into glucose without much effort. Bear in mind that anything that causes an increase of the body's glucose will create an excess of body fat.

Notice that more than 85% of diabetics are overweight. Diabetics are diabetic because their glucose levels are too high and since high levels of glucose force the creation of body fat, more than 85% of them are overweight.

When we eat a doughnut (wheat flour with sugar) the body quickly turns that doughnut into a large amount of glucose in our blood, which sets the scene to gain weight. Those are the mechanics involved in the process of becoming overweight: lots of refined carbohydrates that turn into excess glucose that later become accumulated body fat with the help of the *insulin*[5] hormone.

---

[5] Insulin - a very important hormone that is produced in the pancreas that allows glucose to be transported to the cells to be used as a source of energy

Nothing has contributed more to the rampant obesity epidemic than the excessive consumption of refined carbohydrates. On the contrary, natural carbohydrates like vegetables are excellent foods and don't decrease the metabolism nor contribute to obesity. With the exception of corn and beets, practically all vegetables will help us lose weight and protect our metabolism.

Today, beets are used as the main source of refined white sugar. Because of their high carbohydrate content, they are used to substitute for sugar cane, which used to be used to produce sugar many years ago. On the other hand, few foods are more fattening than corn, for its high content of fructose sugar. Notice that corn and its by-products are used to fatten up pigs, chickens and cattle. Curiously enough, the principal sweetener of carbonated drinks and of many foods in the United States is corn syrup.

There is an economic reality that exists behind all of this. Manufacturers make the most money from producing foods that are carbohydrates. The protein foods (meat, cheese, eggs) are the foods that bring in the smallest profit. Notice that the biggest food manufacturers are companies like *General Foods, Quaker Oats, Nabisco, Kellogg's* and *Nestle.* Look at what they manufacture and sell, all of their products are refined carbohydrates: powdered drinks with sugar, cookies, oatmeal, corn flakes, candies, and chocolates. Refined carbohydrates are by far the biggest source of income for the food industry.

So that you have an idea, years ago I read an economic analysis about the corn flakes business of the Kellogg's Company. An economic analyst of agricultural products had calculated that a family size box of corn flakes that was sold in the supermarket at $1.89, by product net weight, was equivalent to only 11¢ in cost of corn. When you took the amount of ounces of corn that a box of

---

by the body. It is the hormone that allows fat to build up in the body when there is an excess of glucose that isn't used by the cells.

corn flakes contained as a base and you added the price that they paid the farmers for their corn, it was 11¢ in value. Now, imagine yourself in a business in which you can convert 11¢ into $1.89 just by adding a cardboard box, sugar, and advertising. That's a great business!

For the same reason you seldom see television commercials that promote protein such as meat, cheese, or eggs. Protein foods are not profitable enough to justify the big advertising budgets that refined carbohydrates command. This is also why most fast food restaurants offer some type of "make it bigger offers" where they give you an increased proportion of refined carbohydrates (sugary soft drinks, French fries, sweet desserts), never more of the protein such as meat.

It's not that the food manufacturers are bad people. It's that they are good business people! Refined carbohydrates are the big money makers; therefore, they are what all these companies promote. And at the same time, they are what promote the epidemic of weight and obesity problems that affects us. The driving force behind all of this is the money motivation.

The important and intelligent thing is not to get angry with the food marketers. The important and intelligent thing to do is to acquire an awareness about the problem and its causes; the excess consumption of refined carbohydrates. The idea is to protect ourselves and to also protect our loved ones, so that they don't turn into victims of ignorance. We all have the responsibility of knowing about this to protect the health of our loved ones.

CARBOHYDRATES ARE ADDICTIVE

Perhaps the most harmful aspect of refined carbohydrates is their strong addictive power. Yes, refined carbohydrates are addictive. When your body has a craving for something, what does it crave? Does it crave meat or cheese? Or does it crave chocolate, candy, ice cream, bread, or cookies? Notice that the body only craves refined carbohydrates. Refined carbohydrates are like a drug for an addict. People that are addicted to carbohydrates can't control themselves. They eat chocolates and hide the wrappers as if they were criminals. They are trapped in an addiction in the same way that someone addicted to cigarettes needs to smoke, or an alcoholic need to drink alcohol. People addicted to refined carbohydrates need their "fix" like a junkie needs a drug and are trapped in their addiction.

The consumption of these refined carbohydrates in excess doesn't only cause an addiction; it also causes a state of acidity in the body that decreases the metabolism. The excess of refined carbohydrates converts to excess glucose in the blood once it has been digested. Part of the excess glucose ferments within the body and turns into lactic acid, which creates an acidic state that reduces oxygen and decreases the metabolism.

None of this happens when a person eats vegetables or when they eat fruits in moderation. What has changed the most in the last 50 years and has brought our population to an epidemic of weight and obesity problems are the factors of widespread availability and aggressive marketing of thousands of canned, frozen and bagged products that are refined carbohydrates. If we add this to the explosive growth of fast food restaurants that sell primarily refined carbohydrates (French fries, carbonated beverages with sugar, white bread, ice cream) we can then understand the origin of the large quantity of people that today claim to have a "slow metabolism" and that have obesity problems.

On the other hand, there are liquids that because of their high sugar content create an excessive blood glucose level and thus have the effect of causing weight problems and obesity. Milk is an example. Cow milk is very high in its natural sugar, *lactose*. Lactose is a very potent natural sugar that for some people that want to lose weight, it is an obstacle. In fact, lactose is such a potent sugar that it is what drug dealers use to "cut" (dilute) heroin and reduce costs. Years ago, street dealers discovered that if they mixed heroin with *lactose* they would profit more from their drug businesses. Since *lactose* is such a powerful sugar that has the capability of increasing the effects of heroin (addicts call it "the kick"), it is ideal to mix it with heroin for that same reason.

I have met various "milk addicts" within the obese people that I have worked with. They are people that "need" to drink milk in order to feel good because they have already created an addictive relationship with the *lactose* in the milk. Because the majority of the people don't know about these attributes of milk and the fact that the milk industry does an excellent job in promoting their product as a good source of calcium and all kinds of other good things, people feel satisfied with their decision to purchase low fat milk under the belief that it will help them to lose weight. They don't realize that it is the *lactose* in the milk, which makes them gain weight.

For diabetics milk is especially bad. There are various books that mention the harmful effects that milk has on diabetics and on non-diabetics. Books like, *"Don't Drink Your Milk!"* written by Doctor Frank A. Oski.

In my case, I like to drink coffee with milk in the morning. I figure if I use just a little milk, and only for my coffee, I'm not doing myself much harm. Usually I use heavy cream, which is milk fat and is low in carbohydrates, or I use half & half, which is half milk, half cream. I avoid milk in any other liquid form throughout the day.

Refined carbohydrates have another effect that is devastating to your state of mind, your emotions and your enthusiasm for life. Notice that refined carbohydrates cause sleepiness and make you feel tired. After an overdose of sugar and flour (pies, cakes, cookies, doughnuts, etc.) we feel an intense desire to sleep. Refined carbohydrates cause sleepiness. Mothers know this and that is why they give their babies a bottle of milk with sugar, honey or oats when they wake up and cry during the night. The carbohydrates (lactose, honey, sugar, oats, etc.) in the milk make the baby sleepy and induce him to fall asleep so that the parents too can get some sleep.

People that consume a lot of refined carbohydrates are always tired and have a lack of enthusiasm. Their emotions are also affected, because when a person is weak and lacks energy or is tired, they also become intolerant or bad tempered. People who are addicted to carbohydrates tend to have serious hormonal imbalances in their bodies, which in turn produce unstable mental and emotional states. Yes, what we eat does impact our emotions and attitudes because it affects our hormonal system.

The addiction to refined carbohydrates, besides being the cause of weight problems and obesity, is even the cause of depression for some people. Doctors know that people that suffer from hypothyroidism [6] also suffer from depression, insomnia, constipation, and difficulty with weight loss as well as cold hands and feet, among other things. This happens because the thyroid glands produce hormones that control the body's metabolism, as

---

[6] Hypothyroidism - a condition in which the thyroid gland doesn't produce enough of the hormones that control the metabolism and body temperature. This condition is characterized by symptoms like: depression, hair loss, coldness in extremities, constipation, dry skin, difficulty slimming down, constant fatigue, digestive problems and frequent infections.

well as its temperature. When the metabolism is affected, it also affects all of the body's processes and a hormonal imbalance occurs that produces all of these symptoms.

A recent scientific discovery showed that the excess of refined carbohydrates turns into excess glucose (sugar in the bloodstream) which then forces the body to produce an excess of the hormone *insulin* and this hormone at the same time interferes with the hormones of the thyroid glands and brings with it all of the signs of hypothyroidism, including depression. People that are addicted to refined carbohydrates then start to have problems with their thyroid because their bodies produce an excess of *insulin* that interferes with the hormones produced by the thyroid.

Hormones compete against each other for what are called the "cell receptors". Cell receptors could be compared to "doorways" into the cells. When a certain hormone dominates the internal environment of your body, like what happens when an excess of insulin is produced, the dominant hormone blocks the receptors and the other hormones have to wait and can't produce their intended effect upon the cells. An excess of insulin in the body due to an excess of carbohydrate consumption will interfere with the function of the thyroid.

In the human body the only desirable state is that of a balance between the different hormones. When one hormone dominates the environment, the other hormones are impeded from doing their work and this contributes to having a "slow metabolism" condition. This is the case with the excess of *insulin* imposed on our bodies produced by our typical diet of refined carbohydrates

I don't want to exaggerate this topic, but the next time you see someone depressed looking for an escape in food, watch and it is certain that what they will want to eat will be sugar, flour, chocolate or some other sugary food. Refined carbohydrates and depression go hand in hand.

In order to recover your metabolism, it is necessary to take total control of your body and this means that you cannot continue on with addictions that control you. An addiction, by definition, is a condition in which a person obeys the impulses of their body since they have lost control of their body. One of the successful techniques of the NaturalSlim system is the use of the "NATURAL DETOX", which is a period of 48 hours (2 days) in which the person detoxifies their body from the use of refined carbohydrates, completely eliminating them from their diet. Some people are so addicted to carbohydrates that they simply are unable to stop using them, not even for 48 hours unless they receive help in the form of natural supplements that have been developed to help them kick the habit. People who are very addicted to carbohydrates suffer from unpleasant reactions (headaches, diarrhea, muscle pain, etc.) and much anxiety in trying to break this habit if they don't have help from special supplements to break their addiction and calm their hormonal system.

One final note: in reality, there is nothing wrong with having a good piece of pie, a doughnut or bread. It is a matter of establishing if you are controlling the food or if the food is controlling you. The goal then is to achieve a non-addictive state where one is free to use self-determinism about food. To have the ability to freely and without any stress decide if one is going to eat something sweet or some other refined carbohydrate without running the risk of being overpowered by the addictive qualities of these foods.

Food is one of the most exquisite pleasures in life, but you should never let certain foods turn into drugs. There is a difference between "enjoying" and "needing" certain foods. When it comes to food you need to be in control and you can only achieve that by "breaking the habit".

There is a point where you will be free of the addictive influence of refined carbohydrates and you will be able to enjoy them periodically without falling into an addiction cycle. What creates the addiction is the repetitive and continuous use of refined carbohydrates. In other words, if I already feel free from the addiction, I can enjoy them in plain awareness and without the fear of becoming trapped in their addictive effects. It is a matter of having an awareness of the potential addictiveness of these foods and using discipline to be able to enjoy them without becoming trapped or plagued with constant cravings.

A Devastating Effect On Your Health

The excess of refined carbohydrates has had other effects on our population that are less obvious than obesity. It has had a damaging effect on our health in general.

A diet high in refined carbohydrates like bread, pasta, flour, grits, rice, chocolate, candy and starches, like potatoes, causes or aggravates conditions such as: high blood pressure, high triglycerides, and high cholesterol. Diabetics who fail in controlling their consumption of refined carbohydrates never succeed in controlling their diabetes. In addition, it has been proven that there is a direct relation between the excess use of refined carbohydrates and cancer.

People that consume refined carbohydrates in excess force their bodies to create a surplus of glucose in their blood, along with high levels of insulin. Insulin is the hormone that lowers the levels of glucose in your blood and is also the hormone that allows your cells to use glucose as energy.

When you consume an excess of refined carbohydrates your body converts these excess carbohydrates into glucose. An excess of glucose is exactly what doctors refer to as "diabetes". In other words, the excess of glucose puts you on your way to developing or worsening diabetes.

National statistics of childhood and adult diabetes has risen each year for the past 30 years. Every day, childhood obesity is becoming more and more common. It is the excessive consumption of refined carbohydrates that is causing these health problems.

The excess glucose that refined carbohydrates produce forces the body to increase its production of the hormone insulin. This excess insulin then interferes with the thyroid hormone and the person starts to have problems with their thyroid. Problems like depression, irritability, insomnia, weakness, infections and a slow metabolism, among other things. In conclusion, you create a hormonal chaos when you abuse refined carbohydrates.

There is an additional factor that has to do with inflammatory sicknesses in your body. People who consume an excess of refined carbohydrates have more inflammatory conditions in their bodies. In other words, it aggravates inflammatory conditions like migraines, arthritis pain, back pain, heart inflammation, kidney damage and a fatty liver. The diet that has had the best results in lowering inflammatory conditions in the body has been a diet of proteins that are easily digested, like fish, as well as a diet of vegetables and fruits. Vegetables especially have anti-inflammatory effects because they contain substances called "*polyphenols[7]*" that actually block inflammation.

Foods that cause the most inflammation are sugar and refined carbohydrates like doughnuts, cakes, breads and cookies.

On the other hand, because refined carbohydrates have an addictive and calming effect, many people consume them like "drugs" as a refuge during their moments of emotional crisis. Stuffing yourself with doughnuts, ice cream, chocolate or cookies makes your body produce more serotonin, which is a calming and "feel good" substance that is produced in the brain. Antidepressant medications like *Paxil*, *Prozac* and various others work specifically in the brain to increase and reuse serotonin and that produces a calming effect.

The problem is that refined carbohydrates begin affecting our emotional state and create an addictive dependence because of the

---

[7] Polyphenols - are natural plant substances that have antioxidant properties to scavenge free radicals and help the body detoxify. They help maintain a healthy metabolic function.

calming effect that they produce in our bodies. People that are addicted to refined carbohydrates are addicted to food just as drug addicts are addicted to drugs. They <u>have to have</u> their daily "fix" of Coca-Cola, chocolate, candy or some other type of refined carbohydrate. Their emotional health is affected.

It is true; the excessive consumption of refined carbohydrates is making our population sick. Because of the fact that it is damaging our health it is a more serious problem than even the sad reality that each day there are more overweight and obese people in our society.

Dehydration

One of the factors that lower the metabolism the most is dehydration. In other words, lack of water.

Working with thousands of people to help them recover their metabolism, I have seen that a reduced consumption of water has a devastating effect on the metabolism.

The human body is composed mainly of water. It is calculated that your body should be at least 65% water. I have had the opportunity to weigh thousands of people using modern, electronic scales. This type of electronic scale uses a technology that measures the exact amount of water and fat that your body has. This information is much more valuable than just finding out your body weight.

When overweight people are weighed using one of these electronic scales it can be seen that, the more obese a person is, the less the amount of water can be detected in their body. In other words, being overweight really means having a lot of fat and very little water in the body. Thin people's bodies are made up of up to 65% water and those who are obese have a body water content as low as 40%. As a person loses weight the electronic scale detects both an increase in water and a reduction in fat.

The reality is that if a person wants to lose weight, their first step must be to increase their intake of water. Water significantly increases the metabolism. It is logical that it would be that way because when we study the physics of the water molecule, H_2O (two hydrogen atoms and one oxygen atom), we can see that the oxygen atom has a molecular mass 8 times larger than that of the two smaller hydrogen atoms. The water molecule, H_2O, is of similar shape to the cartoon character "*Mickey Mouse*" in which the two hydrogen atoms are Mickey's ears.

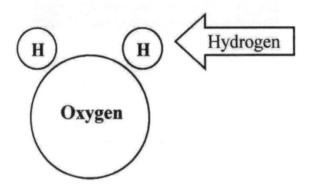

Water, H_2O, is composed of 89% oxygen and only 11% hydrogen when we figure in its molecular mass[8]. When we drink water we are mainly adding oxygen to our bodies. Oxygen is the element that allows the combustion of fat and is what drives the metabolism. Drinking a lot of water is a very effective way to increase your metabolism and to lose weight.

Now, it must be clarified that drinking water and drinking juices or soft drinks is not the same thing. The way that the body functions, if water is just plain water without any flavor, the body sends it to the blood stream and that increases the hydration level and the oxygen availability at the cellular level. If the liquid that we consume has some sort of flavor (soft drinks, juices, coffee, etc.), the body will detect it as food and will send it through the digestive tract, which will not remedy a state of dehydration as effectively or increase the metabolism. Our body knows how to distinguish between what is

---

[8] Molecular mass: all material is composed of atoms. When atoms unite they form molecules. The "molecular mass" refers to the size of the combined atoms that form a molecule.

simply pure water and other liquids (soft drinks, juices, coffee, etc.), which it treats like food.

Drinking soft drinks (Coca-Cola, 7UP, etc.) is one of the best ways to dehydrate the body and decrease the metabolism. Those drinks contain an acid called phosphoric acid, which is what causes the tingling on your tongue when you drink them. The purpose of this acid was to keep the sugar from settling in the bottom of the container and to provide the effervescent and tingling characteristic of soft drinks. Acids, by definition, are substances that reduce oxygen. When we drink a carbonated beverage, even if it is diet cola, the phosphoric acid that it contains reduces a good part of the oxygen that is available in the body and that, at the same time, causes a decrease in the metabolism. I have known obese people whose main action in losing weight was eliminating diet soft drinks from their diet and substituting them with a habit of drinking more water.

When we drink carbonated beverages, diet or not, the body becomes dehydrated. The reason for this is that the human body has to maintain a low level of internal acidity in the blood to be able to survive. Our blood is more alkaline (opposite of acid) than acid because if it weren't, it would repel the oxygen that our cells need. Acids repel oxygen. That is why our blood is more alkaline than acid, so that oxygen can be transported in it. When we drink carbonated beverages with phosphoric acid, our body makes a supreme effort to reduce the level of acids through our urine and this makes the body use part of its water to push out the acids from the soft drinks outside of the body. The more acidic colas or soft drinks we have, the more our body will have to urinate in order to reduce the level of accumulated acids. This worsens the cellular dehydration, as well as reduces the available oxygen to the cells as an effect of the water shortage that is created.

In chemistry you use a pH scale (pH stands for "hydrogen potential") to measure the acidity or alkalinity of substances. On this scale 7.0 is neutral, not acid nor alkaline. Water, for instance, if it is not distilled, is 7.0 in pH on this scale. In other words, it is neutral.

Examples on this scale would be the following:

Substance	pH	
Ammonia	11.0	alkaline
Sea water	8.0	alkaline
Human blood	**7.4**	**alkaline**
Water	7.0	neutral
Milk	6.8	acid
Saliva	6.6	acid
Tomato juice	4.3	acid
Grapefruit juice	3.2	acid
Soft drink cola	**2.5**	**acid**
Vinegar	2.4	acid

It has been calculated that only one 12-ounce can of a carbonated drink (pH 2.5) contains so much acid that it requires as many as 32 glasses of water (8 ounces each) to get the body back to a neutral state (pH 7.0). The sales of soft drinks around the world have been increasing at an accelerated rate in the same way that weight problems, obesity and the so-called "slow metabolism" have increased.

Each time we consume one of those soft drinks we drastically reduce the oxygen in our bodies and force it into a state of internal acidity. Our metabolism suffers the consequences because, in lacking enough oxygen, it finds itself forced to slow down part of its functions.

The human body could be compared to a combustion motor that uses a carbon rich fuel (glucose, a carbohydrate made of carbon, hydrogen and oxygen) and oxygen to generate energy. Like all motors, when the oxygen supply is cut off it reduces its combustion capacity. The combustion capacity of the body is in essence what we call the "metabolism".

People that already have a slow metabolism are always dehydrated. Besides the special electronic scale, like the one that NaturalSlim uses on its members to measure the water in the body, there are various classic indicators of dehydration: dry skin, heartburn, the person practically doesn't sweat, their urine is of a very strong yellow color and with a strong odor of ammonia and they are rarely or never thirsty.

It's an odd but certain fact that the more dehydrated a person is, the more their body will reject water. People that are very dehydrated can't stand drinking water and when they try to drink it they feel like vomiting. In his book *Your Body's Many Cries for Water,* Doctor F. Batmanghelid makes this phenomenon of adaptation of the human body rather clear. When a person is dehydrated the body enters a state of "rationing", which is why their body barely sweats at all. Another thing that a dehydrated body does is that it turns off the sensation of being thirsty as a way to adapt itself to the lack of water. In other words, when you are very dehydrated you simply will not feel thirsty. It has been found that the body takes 3 to 4 days of continuous high-water consumption before reviving the sensation of thirst again. Once the body turns on this sensation of thirst again, the person simply can't stop drinking water, because the thirst sensation that the body produces when it is dehydrated is quite strong.

People that want to increase their metabolism should know that drinking water works. They should also understand that alcohol (wine, beer, liquor) and coffee dehydrate the body. If you go to a bar some time, watch how often the people drinking alcohol have to go to the bathroom. Alcohol dehydrates and acidifies the body, which decreases the metabolism. If you want to lose weight and restore your metabolism, you will have to hydrate your body with a good amount of water while keeping your intake of alcohol and coffee to a minimum.

HOW MUCH WATER DO I NEED TO DRINK?

The amount of water that you should drink each day is relative to the size of your body. The general recommendation that we are used to hearing is that we should drink at least 8-8-ounce glasses of water every day. This is a good recommendation for all of those people who aren't used to drinking enough water, but it isn't exact.

The formula that we have used in NaturalSlim to calculate the recommended daily consumption of water is more exact due to the fact that it takes into consideration the size of the person's body. Logic tells us that a smaller body will need less water than a larger body. A larger body has more capillaries and surface area to hydrate and needs a larger quantity of water. We could say that it is like the difference between the water that you need to clean a small apartment versus the amount needed to clean a house with several rooms.

We calculate the daily water consumption recommended for each person by dividing the weight of the person by the number 16. The result is calculated in 8-ounce glasses of water. For example: if a person weighs 160 pounds and we divide this weight by the number 16 then their daily consumption of water should be 10-8-ounce glasses (160lbs. ÷ 16 = 10 glasses). If a person weighs 240 pounds their recommended water consumption would be 15 glasses a day (240lbs. ÷ 16 = 15 glasses). As you lose weight, you should also reduce your daily intake of water.

For people who find it hard to imagine drinking "8-ounce glasses of water", you should know that you can measure it by bottles of water. Most of the water bottles available everywhere are sold in 16-ounce bottles. This means that each 16-ounce bottle of water is equal to 2-8-ounce glasses of water. So, if a person needs to drink 12-8-ounce glasses of water each day, it would be the same if they were to drink 6 bottles of water every day.

There are different theories as to whether or not you should drink cold water or room temperature water. I don't think it makes any difference. What is important is that each day you drink enough water in order to successfully increase your metabolism.

Drinking enough water is vital in recovering your metabolism. In fact, increasing your consumption of water improves the elimination of toxins from your body and in many cases resolves constipation problems. Water also improves erections for men and the vaginal lubrication of women. So, water can even help improve a couple's sex life and can eliminate the unnecessary use of medications for erectile dysfunction, like Viagra. What happens with people who suffer from asthma is that the majority of them are dehydrated and their asthma attacks disappear when they decide to hydrate their bodies. It should also be known that great majorities of people that suffer from heartburn and acid reflux have this problem because they are dehydrated. When these people decide to drink sufficient amounts of water and stop drinking soft drinks, generally the heartburn and acid reflux disappear. Drinking enough water really can-do wonders. Within the subject of metabolism, water is our greatest ally.

PROBLEMS WITH THE THYROID GLAND SYSTEM

All humans have a gland that is located in the neck that is shaped like a butterfly with its wings open. This gland is called the thyroid gland and its hormones control your metabolism as well as your body temperature.

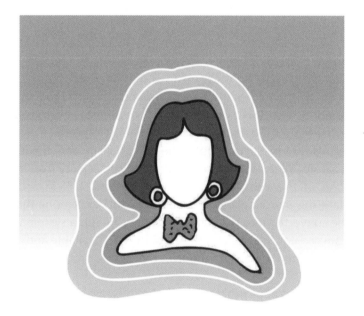

Without going into technical details, we can say that this gland produces a hormone that medicine calls T4. This hormone, T4, is not an active hormone, but more of a storage hormone. It is called T4 because it is made up of 4 atoms. The body, through the action of an enzyme called *deiodinase,* converts the hormone T4 into the T3 hormone, which is an active hormone, not a storage hormone. The T3 hormone is the one that really increases the metabolism and increases the temperature of the body. It is the active hormone.

The T4 hormone would be the equivalent of having petroleum and the T3 would be like having the active and useable product of petroleum, gasoline.

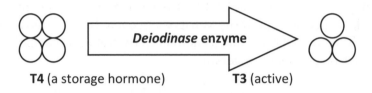

T4 (a storage hormone)   **T3** (active)

There is another hormone that plays a role in this called TSH (*Thyroid Stimulating Hormone*). This is the hormone that the brain produces to request from the thyroid gland a higher production of T4 hormone. The TSH hormone is a "messenger" hormone that carries the brain's orders to the thyroid to tell it to produce more T4, as well as T3, to sustain both the metabolism and the body's temperature. When the brain detects too little activity from the T3 hormone in the cells, it then produces more TSH in order to stimulate the thyroid gland to produce more T4 hormone that can later be converted into the active hormone, T3. It is a system where the brain constantly monitors the amount of T3 available and orders the thyroid gland to produce more T4 through its production of TSH.

People that have problems with their thyroid gland suffer from a condition called hypothyroidism, which is a very common condition and for which there exist various medications, like Synthroid and other brands.

When a person suffers from hypothyroidism they can experience one or several of the following symptoms:

High cholesterol	Difficulty losing weight
Hair loss	Digestive problems
Depression	Dry skin
Constipation	Water retention
Coldness in extremities	Constantly feeling tired
Frequent infections	Memory loss
Lack of interest in sex	Insomnia

If your doctor suspects that you have hypothyroidism, he or she has you do a laboratory test to measure the quantities of T4, T3 and TSH in your blood. There are levels that are considered "normal" for each one of these hormones. Knowing the levels of each hormone allows the doctor to determine which medication will be necessary to correct the situation. Unfortunately, the tests are not infallible, and some experts say that nearly 50% of these tests fail to detect thyroid problems.

Having worked with thousands of overweight and obese people for more than 20 years, I have to agree with these experts that the thyroid hormone laboratory tests are not fail-proof. I have known thousands of people that have all the hypothyroid symptoms and yet their lab tests say they are not hypothyroid. The fact that hypothyroidism doesn't always show in the lab tests is the reason why Dr. Broda Barnes titled his bestseller book "*Hypothyroidism: The Unsuspected Illness*".

It is also important to know that many people that have high cholesterol in reality have a problem with their thyroid that they don't know about. Before the thyroid tests existed that could measure the levels of T4, T3 and TSH in the blood, doctors knew that a person had thyroid problems if they found that their cholesterol was too high, and they knew the person didn't have a diet high in cholesterol. Having high cholesterol could be the clear indicator of the deficient functioning of the thyroid gland.

One of the main signs of hypothyroidism is its tendency to cause weight problems and obesity. People with hypothyroidism find it almost impossible to lose weight because their metabolism is extremely slow since it is their thyroid gland that controls their metabolism. If there is little production of the T3 hormone there will be very little *movement* at the cellular level and the person will have a slow metabolism. What's more, there are people whose laboratory tests reflect "normal" levels of the T3 hormone and yet they have an extremely slow metabolism because, for some reason, their T3 hormone isn't completely active and it is as if it were a defective T3 hormone.

The true energizing action of the T3 hormone happens at the cellular level. The laboratory test measures the amounts of T4 and T3 hormones in the blood but, yet it is not in the blood where the T3 hormone has its energizing effect, it is at the body's cells. Presently there are no tests that can measure the effect that the T3 hormone has on your cells. As a result, the laboratory tests that measure the thyroid hormones in your blood can be of help because they provide a sort of "estimate", but they don't always reflect the truth in all cases. Many people that have extremely slow metabolisms are having problems with the proper functioning of their thyroid hormones. However, their thyroid laboratory tests are reflecting that "everything is ok", while the person continues feeling depressed, having insomnia, experiencing weakness, being overweight and with all of the other potential signs of hypothyroidism.

Oddly enough, hypothyroidism affects 8 women for every 1 man that has this condition. In other words, it is a condition that primarily affects women. Women with hypothyroidism feel weak, tired, and overweight, depressed and sometimes have lost interest in sex. It is a condition that causes many divorces and the saddest part is that in many cases these people go on without knowing that they have a thyroid problem. In his book "*Hypothyroidism: The Unsuspected Illness*", Dr. Broda O. Barnes estimates that about half of the people who suffer from hypothyroidism have not had their condition detected by the traditional laboratory tests that doctors use. So, these people keep on feeling fat, depressed, and weak while their doctor tells them "everything is fine with your thyroid".

In the years that I've worked with thousands of women that wanted to lose weight and restore their metabolism I have had to learn to detect the "subclinical hypothyroidism" that laboratory tests don't detect. I had the luck of discovering the information that Doctor Broda Barnes and Doctor Denis Wilson published in each of their books covering this subject. These two doctors, more than being just doctors, have been brilliant researchers that knew to look past laboratory tests. Both of these doctors cared genuinely about their patients and they both gave more credibility to their patient's symptoms and complaints than to the laboratory test results. In this crazy whirlwind that we call life, it isn't always easy to find a doctor that really listens and observes his or her patients. Economic pressures and time constraints that have been imposed on our doctors by health insurance companies have certainly made us lose part of the quality and time for communication that should exist between the doctor and his patient. As a result, many of our doctors have lost the ability and willingness to have a conversation with their patient to see if the thyroid laboratory test results, in reality, coincide with the symptoms that their patient has. So, they have stopped observing the patient and have substituted it with interpreting what the laboratory analysis says.

According to doctors Broda Barnes and Denis Wilson, approximately 50% of laboratory tests that detect problems with the thyroid gland system gives what they call a "false negative". A "false negative" means that it is "false that there are no problems with the thyroid when in reality there are". Thus, many people who have problems with their thyroid never find out about it.

The thyroid laboratory tests are not reliable. Dr. Barnes was aware that diagnosing thyroid disease by the currently popular blood tests was seriously flawed, missing most of the persons who really are hypothyroid. This is a real disgrace since most people who are hypothyroid are told that "everything is ok with your thyroid hormones" while at the same time being affected by a multitude of hypothyroid symptoms and while also having a "slow metabolism".

The thyroid gland controls the metabolism. When there are problems or defects with the functioning of this gland, the metabolism is affected. Also, when any of these processes that allow your hormones to reach the cells in your body to stimulate and speed up the metabolism fails, chaos is created in your body and that is what is called a "slow metabolism".

The thyroid gland is very sensitive to stress. In fact, stress affects this gland the most. The majority of women, who have problems with their thyroid, start to have problems with it right after some highly emotional or painful traumatic event. Some examples are after going through a bad divorce or after a painful and stressful childbirth. An automobile accident or losing a loved one can also cause thyroid problems. All in all, it is a gland that is seriously affected by stress.

On the other hand, the thyroid gland has specific needs for certain nutrients, vitamins and minerals that, if lacking, will impede its production of hormones. In order to function adequately, the thyroid cannot have any deficiencies of any of the following substances: iodine, zinc, magnesium, copper, manganese, selenium and the amino acid L-Tyrosine. If your body has a shortage of any of these needed substances, the thyroid could be affected, and it could be a cause of hypothyroidism with the resulting "slow metabolism".

If you suffer from a slow metabolism, and you also have several of the symptoms of hypothyroidism that were listed before, you might suspect that there are problems with your thyroid gland. The laboratory tests that exist are of some help, but they are not always 100% correct in detecting a hypothyroid condition.

YOUR TEMPERATURE SAYS IT ALL

It is easy to get distracted by the technical details of laboratory exams and the sophisticated technology of X-rays and electromagnetic equipment. Sometimes we have all of the obvious signs right in front of us in a situation and we choose not to see them. This is the case with problems with the thyroid gland, in which the majority of our doctors have come to rely solely on laboratory exams and have stopped observing the most obvious symptoms. There are many people who suffer from thyroid problems and as a result, they also suffer from depression. This happens, even though their laboratory tests show that "everything is fine with the thyroid" and yet the person feels horribly bad. When the laboratory test does not detect that the person is hypothyroid many times the person will be accused of imagining conditions that he or she does not have and treated as a hypochondriac (one that complain of having sicknesses that do not really exist). The majority of doctors have come to believe that the laboratory tests that measure the thyroid hormones are infallible and that it is the patient that exaggerates conditions that they really don't have.

Luckily, we have doctors that do listen, like Dr. Barnes and Dr. Wilson. Both of these doctors use the most basic test to detect thyroid problems for their diagnoses: BODY TEMPERATURE. Since your thyroid controls your body temperature, when it isn't functioning properly, your body temperature directly reflects it. The body of a person whose thyroid has hormone production problems or T4 to T3 conversion problems will be colder than those who do not have thyroid problems. The thyroid gland is like a thermostat for the human body, when it isn't functioning your body feels colder than normal.

The normal temperature for all human bodies is and should be 98.6 Fahrenheit or 37 C on the centigrade scale. Any temperature that is at or below 97.8 F or at 36.5 C or below, shows that there are problems with the thyroid gland system. The temperature of the human body can vary some decimals in degrees throughout the course of a day, but when it goes down to 97.8 F or less or 36.5 C or less, a good part of the metabolism processes are going to be affected.

The human body's normal temperature is a very narrow range. For example, a body temperature that on the average is 98.4 F or 98.8 F could be ok. But, when the body's temperature starts to drop closer to 98.0 F it generally means trouble the same way that when it goes up to 99.0 F we can call it a "slight fever". The body's tolerance for temperature variations is indeed narrow.

Within the human body there are over 500 different enzymes[9] whose function is to achieve biochemical changes in the hormones, the cells and the blood. Enzymes are proteins that are very sensitive to temperature. Some enzymes depend on the body maintaining a body temperature of 98.6 F (37.0 C) or a temperature very close to it in order to function. When the body cools down as a result of thyroid problems, many of the processes of the metabolism are interrupted and this is what causes the symptoms of depression, coldness in the extremities, obesity, insomnia and other symptoms.

An effective and simple way to know if your thyroid is functioning well is to take your body's temperature with a glass thermometer. The temperature should be taken at least 3 times

---

[9] Enzymes - Enzymes are proteins that participate in changes and transformations of other substances. For example, there is an enzyme that transforms and turns cholesterol into the hormone *estrogen*. There are different enzymes that are used to digest fats, proteins and carbohydrates. There are also enzymes in the body whose main function is to disable toxic substances that penetrate the body. Some enzymes break the bonds that exist between food atoms and this frees the energy that the food contains. There are enzymes involved in all of the body's processes.

throughout the day, and at least 1 hour after having eaten. You could do this for two days (6 measurements) and then your results should be averaged to find out your average body temperature. If the average temperature is equal to or less than 97.8 F or equal to or less than 36.5 C, there are problems with your thyroid. If your body's temperature is low, you will also have a "slow metabolism". So, taking your temperature serves as a way to find out if you have a "slow metabolism" or a normal one.

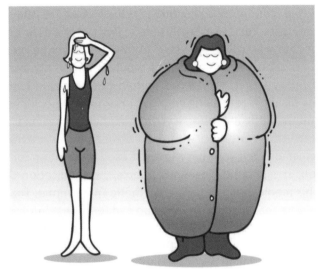

A SLOW METABOLISM RESULTS IN A COLD BODY TEMPERATURE

Your body temperature reflects how slow or how fast your metabolism goes. People that have a slow metabolism suffer and complain of being cold because in reality their bodies are colder than normal.

Electronic digital thermometers are very fast but are not very precise. Try to use a traditional glass thermometer with mercury or one of the newer non-mercury glass thermometers. These thermometers require between 3 to 4 minutes to correctly record your body's temperature, but they are very exact. You use the temperature of your mouth.

Knowing this temperature data allows you to seek medical help if the temperature consistently shows that your thyroid is not working properly. You can have some difficulty finding a doctor that is willing and ready to listen to you and help if your thyroid laboratory tests don't show that you are hypothyroid. Don't give up, there are still some doctors that have clinical orientation (of observing symptoms) and that are willing to provide you with a prescription for thyroid hormones[10] as a "test dosage". I know that this is the case because I had the same problem of having a hypothyroid condition that didn't reflect itself in the thyroid laboratory tests. Yet, I was finally able to find (after 3 different visits) a doctor that was willing to listen to me and prescribe me a "test dosage" to allow me to see if they would improve my symptoms. When I finally began to use the thyroid hormone the continuous tiredness disappeared, along with the insomnia, the coldness in my limbs and the difficulty losing weight that I had always had.

I must also tell you that the most used medication for thyroid conditions is Synthroid. For many people this medication does not work. This medication contains a synthetic T4 hormone. That is why many people that use this medication can feel some improvement, but it doesn't really help them to increase their metabolism if the person's body has a problem with converting the T4 hormone to the active hormone T3. If you remember the explanation about the thyroid hormone, you will see that T4 is the "storage hormone", not the active hormone. The active hormone is T3, which the body extracts from T4 with the help of the enzyme *deiodinase*. The problem is that many people have slow metabolisms because they also have a CONVERSION problem in which the T4 hormone doesn't efficiently convert to T3 (active hormone), and therefore, the metabolism keeps lacking energy. So, putting more T4 (Synthroid) into your body doesn't necessarily resolve the problem of having a slow metabolism if the body has a problem in converting the T4

---

[10] Thyroid hormones: refers to the hormones that are produced by the thyroid gland.

hormone to the T3 hormone, which is the active hormone at the cellular level.

There are medications for the thyroid that come from natural sources, like Armour[11], which is a thyroid hormones complex that is extracted from the thyroids of pigs and contains both T4 and T3. Many people who have been struggling with their weight for years have asked their doctor to switch them from using Synthroid (synthetic T4 hormone) to using Armour (natural T4 with T3 hormones) and have finally been able to lose weight. There are websites like www.drugstore.com where you can order Armour with your doctor's prescription. The most difficult thing is, if you suspect that your thyroid isn't working properly, and your thyroid test come back "normal", is to get a friendly doctor that is willing to prescribe you a "test dosage" to observe the betterment it could produce in you.

Some doctors believe that the temperature test is unscientific and will rely solely on standard blood tests. If your lab tests come back "normal" and your body's cold temperature and your symptoms indicate that you have a thyroid problem, you might have to do a lot of searching to find a doctor that is willing to look deeper than the standard blood tests. Doctors that believe in the value of what is called the "basal temperature test" (taking the body's temperature) will give you a prescription for thyroid hormones and start to increase the dosage very gradually in what is called "titration[12]". In other words, they gradually adjust the dosage of the medicine until the desired effects are noticed. Not every doctor is knowledgeable in this area.

The metabolism is all about movements. The movements use energy and produce HEAT. The more movement there is, the more heat there will be; the less movement there is, the more coldness

---

[11] Aside from Armour there are other natural thyroid hormones sold under the Westhroid or Naturethroid brands.
[12] Titration- the process of gradually adjusting the dose of a medication until the desired effect is achieved

there will be. Notice that if you hold a newborn baby in your arms you will always feel its body warm because of the extensive amount of growth movements that are happening in its young and energetic body. The metabolism of a newborn baby is always fast and therefore feels so warm. On the contrary, notice the temperature of an older person, they will always feel colder to touch. This is because the older person has already lost a good part of its metabolism with age and its body is getting colder and slower. I've worked with overweight and obese people for more than 20 years, and I must admit that I can't help but to feel and estimate the temperature and the metabolism of a person that I've recently met after shaking their hand and feeling the temperature of their body. Your temperature tells it all!

If you have suspected that you have a "slow metabolism" it is possible that the real cause is an undisclosed thyroid problem. This is the time when you should pull out the glass thermometer and find out if your difficulty in losing weight and "slow metabolism" is being caused by hypothyroidism. Not checking your body's temperature will leave you with a mystery because if you happen to be hypothyroid all your efforts to lose weight could end in another failure. So, check your body's temperature and find out for yourself if medical help is needed or not.

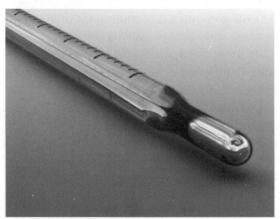

USING A GLASS THERMOMETER WILL HELP YOU KNOW HOW YOUR THYROID GLAND IS DOING

Another interesting piece of information is that nothing affects the thyroid more than stress. That is one of the reasons that it has been discovered that stress makes you gain weight. Like I mentioned before, the conditions of the thyroid that cause a "slow metabolism" affect a total of 8 women for every 1 man affected. In the case of a woman or a man the thyroid can be affected by experiencing some sort of family crisis, an accident, a sickness or a difficult problem. In the specific case of women, the thyroid can be affected mainly after childbirth due to the severe physical and emotional stress that giving birth can have on the bodies of women. Perhaps that is why the majority of women lose their beautiful "newlywed" figure after having a baby; their thyroid is affected.

There are also certain vitamins and mineral deficiencies like zinc, iodine, selenium, magnesium and others that can create problems with the thyroid and can also prevent an efficient conversion from the T4 hormone to the active T3 hormone. In other words, nutrition is also a factor.

In recent years, a huge discovery was made that helped people with thyroid and metabolism problems considerably. The discovery had to do with the properties of organic coconut oil. Organic coconut oil, a natural product, increases your body temperature and your metabolism and helps people that have had difficulties in losing weight as a result of having a "slow metabolism". Taking a dose of this natural oil every day has allowed many people, who before lost weight very slowly, to now lose weight at a more satisfactory speed. Organic coconut oil contains a saturated fat called "medium chain triglycerides" which notably and measurably increases your body temperature and metabolism. In fact, in taking a daily dose of organic coconut oil, you can then take your temperature and see the increase of your body temperature. The increase of your body temperature also causes an increase of your metabolism and more ease in losing weight.

In past years, there had been a lot of erroneous and negative information about coconut oil in the media. In another chapter in this book we will analyze more thoroughly the topic of organic coconut oil and the scientific data that supports it.

For the moment what is important to know is that your temperature tells it all!

STRESS MAKES YOU GAIN WEIGHT

Everyone talks about stress. But, what is stress? Stress is a reaction. It is the reaction that our mind and body have when our survival is threatened.

Any threat, real or imaginary, unexpected noise or movement, accident, fall, blow, sudden change in temperature, worry about present or the future, possible loss of something or of a loved one, obstacle or unexpected problem, danger to one's security, a health problem or a sickness will all cause a stress reaction. Stress is an instantaneous reaction that can become so violent that it causes a heart attack.

Generally, stress doesn't get to the point of causing a heart attack, but it does create a state of GENERAL ALARM so extreme that our entire hormonal and nervous system is affected. Each cell in our body is affected by the reaction we call stress. It is an effect that is definitely cumulative. You only need to notice how worn out and tired a person looks who has recently lost a loved one in order to see how stress affects the entire body in a thousand and one ways.

On the other hand, after having experienced a state of severe stress, the body and mind take some time to go back to being calm and regaining the inner peace. Stress is a factor of mental instability that causes a state of DISORDER throughout the entire body.

Some people live in a state of stress that is so continuous that they can't distinguish whether they feel stress or not. When someone is stressed out on a routine basis they find it difficult to be fully aware of the fact that they are living a stress filled life. For example, a person who finds himself or herself forced to work in a job in which he or she is mistreated will feel continuously stressed while at their job. The same thing happens when a person experiences problems with their family or with a romantic partner and they have to live with it day after day. When stress becomes part of our daily life we grow accustomed to it and sometimes accept it as "normal".

Besides the observable damage that stress can cause to your body and health, there is a factor that is measurable. It is a hormonal factor. When you are stressed your body produces an excess of the hormone *cortisol*[13]. This hormone, *cortisol,* is called the "stress hormone" because your body produces it when you experience a stressful situation.

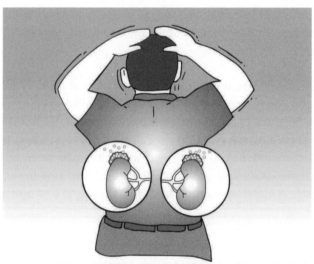

STRESS PROVOKES THE PRODUCTION OF CORTISOL

---

[13] Cortisol is a hormone produced by the adrenal glands (gland on top of our kidneys). It is often referred to as the "stress hormone" as it is involved in the response to stress. Among other effects it increases blood pressure, blood sugar levels and also lowers the body's immune (defense) system.

The *cortisol* hormone is produced in the adrenal glands that are found above each of our two kidneys.

The *cortisol* hormone is a vital part of our internal ALARM system. Our body produces this hormone with the purpose of using it to handle any emergency that is detected in our environment. It is a hormone that prepares the body for "fight or flight". It was designed by nature to allow us to overcome a dangerous situation using our best physical and mental resources. That is why when we produce the hormone *cortisol* in response to a stressful situation our body responds to this hormone by producing some internal changes that help us better survive the supposed danger or threat. These are internal changes like raising the blood pressure and greatly increasing the level of glucose (blood sugar, the body's fuel) to higher levels. The glucose level is increased so that the cells have enough energy available to fight or flee.

If the source of stress were a tiger that was chasing us down to tear us to shreds, all of this excess glucose that the *cortisol* put in our blood stream would be consumed by our efforts in running to get away from the tiger and there wouldn't be a surplus of glucose after the period of stress. The problem is that when the source of the stress is for a short period of time, say some bad news, the glucose levels increase due to the *cortisol*, but the excess glucose that is not taken in by the cells is turned into fat to be stored. Glucose is the principal source of energy of all of the cells in our body, but when it isn't used and there is excess, the body turns it into fat to store it, as a source of energy for future use. Thus, stress produces an excess of glucose in the blood through the action of *cortisol* and this excess of glucose ends up being converted to fat that is then stored into our waistline, hips and abdomen. Yes, stress definitely makes us gain weight.

It must be said that the source of stress could be external or internal. With this I want to say that it really is true that bad news (something external to the body) causes stress that produces large amounts of *cortisol*. It is also true that an internal infection or sickness in our bodies produces large amounts of *cortisol* because our body perceives the situation as dangerous and reacts to it with an increase in its production of cortisol. Example: people that have internal bacterial, viral, fungal (yeasts) or parasitic infections in their body will see that many times they gain weight without having eaten more than usual mostly due to the increase of *cortisol* in their body. Any stress, external or internal, will make your body produce more *cortisol*, lower your metabolism and make you gain weight. Even having the wrong marital partner can force your body to produce excessive *cortisol* and that will make it difficult if not impossible for you to lose weight.

The *cortisol* produced by stress, has other negative effects like causing memory or concentration loss. That's why when we are stressed out we can't think clearly. *Cortisol* also weakens the immune system, which is our internal defense system. People under stress become sick much easier and more frequently. *Cortisol* also affects our digestive system and can produce an over acidic state in our stomach, as well as cause stomach ulcers. Stress produces *cortisol*, and an excess of *cortisol* has the ability of weakening all of our organs and cells. In addition, it has been seen that stress increases the internal acidity of the body and lowers the oxygen levels, which aggravates the functioning of the metabolism even more.

People that live in conditions of stress from work or family gain weight much easier because their levels of *cortisol* tend to be excessively high. *Cortisol* increases the glucose in your blood by giving orders to the liver to use its glucose reserves and to deposit it into the blood stream to handle the emergency of the state of ALARM, which it believes itself under. When a stressful situation occurs and the *cortisol* successfully uses our liver glucose reserve we automatically feel hungry, especially for sweet foods and those that are a source of glucose like carbohydrates: bread, flour, chocolate, pasta, etc. So, it's not just that stress makes you gain weight; it also makes you feel hungry. That's why a person that feels depressed by a personal or family problem many times seeks solace in the refrigerator.

There are natural strategies available to use to control the harmful effects of stress. There are also natural supplements that can control the excessive production of the *cortisol* hormone to prevent the stress that makes us gain weight and makes us hungry. When you cleanse your body of the yeasts and parasites you also lower your internal stress levels and lower your *cortisol* levels. This is how many people have lost weight; after having done a cleansing program of yeasts and parasites using natural supplements. Anything that reduces stress increases our metabolism and helps us in losing weight. A better job, a good partner, an entertaining hobby and enjoyable vacations are all successful and positive influences to increasing your metabolism and reducing stress.

Stress produces *cortisol* and it was also discovered that *cortisol* interferes with the thyroid gland, which lowers the metabolism. So, this is another way in which stress lowers the metabolism, because it interferes with our thyroid.

The best way to find out if stress is affecting you too much and to see if it is one of the reasons that you are experiencing a slow metabolism is to take note of your quality of sleep. Since the *cortisol* hormone is an ALARM hormone it creates a strong state of ALERT in the body that doesn't allow us to sleep peacefully. To the body's cells *cortisol* is like an urgent warning of impending danger. *Cortisol* excites the cells and puts them in a state of ALERT, thus you won't sleep well when under stress.

When there is too much *cortisol* in our blood it makes it difficult for us to get sleep. On the other hand, the excess *cortisol* makes us get a different kind of sleep; a sleep quality that is called "light sleep" and we wake up feeling tired in the morning. Sleep has different stages, which determine its quality and restfulness. The *cortisol* produced while under stress keeps the cells in a constant state of ALARM and impedes what is called the "deep sleep" stage, which is the most restful and invigorating sleep for the body. It is the state of ALARM created by *cortisol* that steals our quality of sleep. Who can sleep peacefully when feeling in danger?

Throughout the years I have learned never to ask people if they are under a lot of stress that doesn't allow them to lose weight. I realized that some people live under such a constant state of stress that they can't distinguish if they are stressed out or not anymore. Because they are always under stress they consider it a "normal" state. That is why the only question I ask a person, in order to find out if they have too much *cortisol* in their body, as a result of stress, is: how well do you sleep? The answer to this question tells me what I want to know in relation to the level of stress that the person is experiencing.

Something additional that we know about *cortisol* and about stress is that when we experience a condition of stress our levels of *cortisol* dramatically increase and remain in our body for more than 8 hours after the incident before going back to normal levels. So, the effects of high levels of *cortisol* are long lasting. However, when we do moderate exercise (walking, swimming) for 30 to 45 minutes our body eliminates huge amounts of *cortisol* through the liver and this also makes the state of ALARM produced by *cortisol* to go away much earlier. That's why many people find that if they have had a very stressful day, they will have a very difficult time sleeping unless they do a bit of exercise before going to bed. Exercise helps us get good sleep because it lowers the level of *cortisol* that is in our bloodstream.

Your metabolism will be affected greatly by the *cortisol* hormone that it generates during stressful moments. All of this is enough to help you realize that your lifestyle is very much related to the condition of your metabolism and to the general state of your health.

BAD DIGESTION

Something noticeable in people that are overweight or obese is that many times they suffer from one or several of the following digestive problems: heartburn, acid reflux, intestinal gases, flatulence or constipation. In general, these are digestive problems that medications can't completely eliminate.

Another one of the factors that lowers the metabolism is bad digestion. This happens because the cells in our body can't use the foods that we eat, unless the digestive process reduces them to the smallest molecular size to guarantee absorption. So, our cells can't use a piece of meat because meat is a protein whose molecule is too big to fit inside a space as small as a cell. What nourishes our body and increases our metabolism isn't what we eat, it is what our body is able to absorb through digestion.

The foods that we eat are composed of tiny molecules and atoms. Unless these foods can be converted into their smallest molecular sizes, they will not be able to be used by the cells. It is a problem of size.

Food starts digesting from the moment our saliva comes into contact with it. Later on, in the stomach, the body uses enzymes and very powerful acids that, when they work properly, succeed in breaking even the toughest foods, such as pork rinds, for example. The digestion later continues throughout the intestines, where the environment turns from acid to alkaline (opposite of acid) and this completes digesting everything that wasn't digested before. Finally, in the last part of the small intestine, nutrients are extracted from the foods already softened and broken down molecularly by the digestive system. The process takes between 12 to 16 hours to complete. When a person suffers from constipation it could take up to 36 hours or more.

One of the most effective ways to increase your metabolism and lose weight is by improving your digestion. There are various aids that work. They are things like:

• Drink a lot of water. Water improves digestion because it eliminates excessive acidity and creates the most effective means of transportation that there is for nutrients, the blood. Many cases of heartburn are simply cases of severe dehydration where the body finds itself impeded from making the alkaline substances that counteract stomach acids because of the water shortage.

• Take digestive enzymes. When a person is already experiencing bad digestion (heartburn, acid reflux, gas), the use of digestive enzyme capsules or tablets with each meal can be a real help in increasing their metabolism. Enzymes help the body digest food completely and then increase the absorption of nutrients which raise the metabolism. There are digestive enzymes for digesting proteins, carbohydrates and fats. Generally, the different types of digestive enzymes come combined in capsules or tablets and you can get them in any natural food store.

• Lower your intake of refined carbohydrates like bread, flour, pasta, rice and sugar. These refined carbohydrates cause an excess of acidity because all of them, when used in excess, turn into a surplus of glucose (blood sugar). When excess glucose accumulates inside of your body it ferments and turns into acids like lactic acid, which increases the acidity in your body and reduces absorption. Many people that suffer from digestive problems see their problems disappear very quickly by reducing the refined carbohydrates in their diet.

• Don't combine foods that don't go well together like for example, fruit and cheese. Vegetables generally go well with meats, eggs and cheese but fruits ferment when they are combined with proteins like meat, cheese or eggs. Everything that ferments during digestion will produce gases. Furthermore, our body can't use foods that ferment

94

during digestion and thus they tend to lower the metabolism as opposed to increasing it.

When food creates gases inside our body it is only because there is something fermenting or decomposing. A healthy digestion doesn't produce gases or bad odors.

In my experience I have seen that simply reducing refined carbohydrates and increasing the consumption of water can do miracles. People that do it stop using antacid medications and start enjoying good digestion and are given a more agile metabolism that helps them lose weight or maintain their figure.

At times, we tend to think that the solutions to our problems should be complex when, really, we have the remedies right under our noses. If a person suffers from heartburn, ulcers, acid reflux or other digestive problems it will be nearly impossible to lose weight. The solution could be as simple as avoiding soft drinks (examples: Coca Cola, Pepsi-Cola, 7-Up) that are acids, increasing the consumption of water and reducing refined carbohydrates. In a short time, the person will experience a marked improvement.

In principle, everything that makes digestion difficult will also have the effect of reducing our metabolism and everything that makes digestion more efficient will speed up our metabolism. Bad digestion will produce bad absorption of nutrients. Bad absorption takes the body to a very low state of cellular energy. This low energy state contributes to what is called a "slow metabolism". In order to lose weight and speed up your metabolism it is essential that you improve your digestive process.

ENEMY SUBSTANCES

Everything that we eat has some effect on our body. This includes all foods, medications, preservatives, dyes and any other substance that is part of what we eat and drink.

Some of the substances that we consume regularly are harmful to our metabolism and make it slower. This is the case with polyunsaturated[14] oils like corn, soybean and vegetable oil, which we commonly buy in the supermarket and that are regularly used as ingredients in prepared or canned food. The same happens with canola oil, which we used to recommend 15 years ago as "good for the metabolism". Now, modern science, by improving its technology, has discovered that canola[15] oil is a very harmful and toxic to the thyroid and health in general, therefore, we do not recommend it anymore.

Different researchers have proven that polyunsaturated oils like corn, soybean and vegetable oil interfere with the function of the thyroid gland. Until a few years ago, the most harmful oil to the thyroid gland was the soybean oil and now the canola oil joins it. Since the thyroid gland controls the body's metabolism these oils have the effect of lowering the metabolism. This is why it is recommended that you use oils like coconut oil to fry and olive oil

---

[14] Polyunsaturated - oils and fats are made up of molecules of carbon, hydrogen and oxygen atoms. When all of the carbon atoms of oil are joined with hydrogen atoms it is then called a saturated fat (pig fat, coconut oil, etc.). If there are carbon atoms that aren't joined to hydrogen atoms, then the oil is polyunsaturated oil (corn oil, vegetable oil, etc.).

[15] Canola: a type of vegetable oil that is extracted from the rapeseed.

for all other cooking that doesn't require frying. The one limitation that olive oil has is that it can't take much heat and that is why it isn't recommended as frying oil.

In order to protect your metabolism, it is necessary to avoid poly-unsaturated oils like corn, canola, soybean and vegetable oil.

Since we are talking about oils, it is also appropriate for us to also touch on the subject of fats. We have been bombarded by the media with a massive advertising campaign, to warn us about the dangers of cholesterol and, also, to sell us "cholesterol-free" products. From that anti-cholesterol campaign was born the bright idea of substituting butter, a fat that contains cholesterol, with a manmade fat called margarine. At first, it seemed like a good idea.

What they didn't tell us is that ALL margarines contain a high content of "trans fatty acids", which are very harmful to our health and also lower our metabolism. Margarine is an industrial product that is created in a very chemically violent process. This process is called "hydrogenation", which consists of taking any polyunsaturated liquid oil (corn, soybean, sunflower, vegetable) and heating it to very high temperatures, and while putting a high voltage current in it and at the same time also pumping hydrogen gas into it in order to get the oil to turn solid. When the hydrogen unites with the oil molecules the oil turns into a white greasy substance that you can spread. It goes from liquid to solid.

Trans-fatty acids are fat molecules that have been damaged and deformed by intensive heat and the electric currents used in the processing. They are fat molecules that have lost their normal molecular shape and have been left in a deformed shape. As a result, the body treats it as if it were toxic because it doesn't recognize it as edible and it doesn't allow it to be used as a nutrient for the cells. There is a new federal regulation from the Food and Drug Administration (FDA) that is gradually going into effect. It requires manufacturers to label their foods stating the amount of trans-fatty acids contained in each food. This is what consumer groups have achieved by putting pressure on the FDA to require food manufacturers to reveal the content of these molecularly altered fats. In some cases, margarine can be made have up to 40% in trans-fatty acids.

Manufacturers of margarine know that we wouldn't buy that white greasy substance because it doesn't look very appetizing. However, they have an excellent marketing technique. What they do is mix the margarine with a yellow dye ("yellow #5") so that it looks like the color of butter and so that it appears more appetizing like butter. If we were to see the true white, greasy color, it wouldn't occur to us to spread it on bread, because it is disgusting.

Contrary to what the consumers of margarine are made to think, there are various studies that reflect that the consumption of margarine raises their cholesterol and also increases the incidence of heart problems. If you decide to improve your metabolism and lose weight you should avoid consuming margarine. Butter, on the other hand, is a saturated fat that contains cholesterol, but is a fat that the body can use naturally and that doesn't contain the trans-fatty acids that are harmful to your health. Butter is yellow because the cow and God decided it to be that way, it doesn't have dyes. Butter will help you lose weight; margarine will make you gain weight.

On the other hand, soybean has been promoted on a grand scale by the biggest agriculture companies and by the food industry as something that is "healthy". The reality is that the studies that have been used to demonstrate the benefits of soybean are studies that were done in Japan where the soy is fermented (examples: soy sauce, tofu). The natural process of fermentation used in the orient destroys the thyroid blocking properties of soy and makes the soy healthy for us. Our reality in the west is that the soy is industrially processed, without fermentation, by using chemicals. That's why the soy that we are sold isn't healthy for us. The soy that is sold in our stores, whose preparation process doesn't include fermentation, contains compounds called "goitrogens [16] " that reduce the functioning of the thyroid. These compounds interfere with the mineral iodine that is essential to the proper functioning of the thyroid gland. I have seen many vegetarians that have started to have obesity problems probably because of their high consumption of soy in its different forms. If you suffer from a slow metabolism, avoid soy.

Many studies have revealed the harm that soy can cause. Researchers at the Medical College of Cornell University said that babies who have been fed soy milk formula were more prone to develop thyroid problems. It was also discovered that those babies who are fed with soy had more than double the incidence of diabetes than those babies that were not fed soy.

There is another substance that definitely lowers the metabolism and doesn't help people lose weight. It is the artificial sweetener aspartame that is sold in the supermarket under various commercial brands like *NutraSweet, Equal, Same* and other brand names. This substance, aspartame, lowers the metabolism and creates a desire for sweet foods. This is something that I have closely observed after having worked with more than hundreds of thousands of people within the NaturalSlim weight loss system. If someone who wanted to lose weight ingested some food or drink sweetened with aspartame they either didn't lose weight or they lost weight too slowly. As soon as they eliminated aspartame from their diet they began to lose weight at a faster rate.

On one occasion I tried to convey this information on the NaturalSlim website and we received a legal threat from the manufacturers of aspartame. We decided to remove our opinion from the Internet. At that time, our only other alternative and one

---

[16] Goitrogens: substances that suppress thyroid function. Goitrogens can induce hypothyroidism. Goitrogens work by interfering with the thyroid's uptake of iodine.

that we weren't ready for, was to spend a huge fortune to defend ourselves from the attacks of the lawyers of the manufacturer of aspartame who devoted themselves to threatening all of those people that try to tell the truth about aspartame. Well, the truth is the truth. Aspartame will both lower your metabolism and spike your craving for sweets.

Anyway, if you are interested in protecting your metabolism you are going to have to read the labels so that you can eliminate aspartame from your diet. There are other artificial sweeteners that don't seem to have the same depressing effect on the metabolism that aspartame does. They are other artificial sweeteners like *stevia*, *sucralose* (*Splenda*) and *Acesulfame Potassium (Acesulfame K)* which in my experience allow you to lose weight.

Another substance that is an enemy of the metabolism is fluoride. Fluoride is used in many states in the tap water that we use to cook and bathe. Fluoride is also found in practically all brands of toothpaste. What has been discovered is that fluoride decreases the functioning of the thyroid gland. In fact, in the 1950's, fluoride was used as a medication to lower the production of an over-active thyroid condition. In a clinical study it was demonstrated that a daily dose of only 2.5 to 4.5 milligrams was successful in reducing the production of hormones in the thyroid and it treated hyperthyroidism (excessive production of thyroid hormones). In areas where water contains fluoride, the daily consumption can get up to 6.5 milligrams per day, which can negatively affect your thyroid.

If you are experiencing a slow metabolism you should avoid using toothpaste that contains fluoride. All health food stores offer non-fluoride toothpaste. Your water should be bottled or filtered in some type of filter that guarantees the removal of the fluoride. You should also avoid the fluoride treatments that dentists use to whiten your teeth; you could end up having beautifully white teeth and a severe hypothyroid condition.

In our fight to recover our metabolism, it is vital that we avoid the substances that lower our metabolism.

THE FOOD INTOLERANCES

Just about everyone knows what an allergy is. Allergies are closely connected to itching, mucus, sneezing, headaches and asthma attacks, along with various other effects. In some cases, allergic reactions can be rather dangerous. Like when someone who has a seafood allergy eats something that contains seafood and it causes such a serious allergic reaction that the person must be taken to the hospital.

An allergy is your immune system reacting because for one reason or another it has identified a food or substance (dye, preservative, chemical, protein, etc.) as an "enemy", and it attacks it as such. Allergies are noticed because they cause: swelling, itching, headaches, mucus, etc.

To fully understand the subject of the metabolism we must also touch on the subject of the food intolerances which are different than a regular allergic reaction. Food intolerances are less obvious reactions that the body has to those foods that it doesn't tolerate but that have the effect of also reducing the metabolism. These reactions don't produce strong allergic reactions, like allergies do, because they don't involve the body's immune system. Yet they can stop you from losing weight if you are not aware of their existence. They are reactions to foods that the body rejects. It has been seen that when we consume one of these foods that our body dislikes, the metabolism is lowered, and it makes it difficult or impossible for us to lose weight.

The food intolerances of the body are more difficult to detect than allergies since they don't provoke a visible allergic reaction.

However, if your body ends up being intolerant to any food and you consume it, you will notice how your metabolism becomes stagnant and that won't allow you to lose weight.

In my search for the reasons behind the slow metabolism I discovered that food intolerances really do exist. When we eat any food that our body doesn't like, the metabolism slows down and it makes it impossible for us to lose weight.

In working with thousands of people that wanted to lose weight I have found that the foods that cause the most "intolerances" are corn, soybean and wheat. When your body is "intolerant" to one or several of them and you ingest them, your metabolism becomes stagnant and your body will not get rid of the fat.

Corn is the main source of the sweetener used by the industries that manufacture soft drinks. The sweetener product is called "high fructose corn syrup" or HFCS. For example, Coca-Cola, as well as pretty much every other soft drink, is sweetened with corn syrup. Corn syrup is found in many prepared foods because it is a very economical sweetener and that's why manufacturers prefer it. There are some people that simply cannot lose weight if they consume any product derived from corn because they happen to have intolerance to corn or corn derived products. It has taken me a lot of work to figure this out. Working with thousands of people that wanted to lose weight, I saw that this was the case.

One time I was helping a member of the NaturalSlim system lose weight and I ran into a clear case of intolerance to corn and its derived products. If I hadn't realized that something was stopping the metabolism of this person, he would have failed in his attempt to lose weight.

In researching the causes of a slow metabolism, I have many times had to take the position of a detective. The experience has showed me that when a person is successfully losing weight and then suddenly stops losing weight and becomes stagnant; it is because some factor that affects their metabolism has changed. When I see that something that was working well suddenly stops working, time has trained me to ask, "What changed?" I don't believe in luck, I believe in skill or ability.

In this member's case, he had a situation in which he had been losing 2 to 3 pounds continually each week. This man had already lost more than 40 pounds and was trying to lose the last 20 pounds of fat. It was satisfying to see him every week because he always told us how good he felt, and the truth was that every week he looked better physically than he had the week before.

However, after several weeks that he had been losing weight, he suddenly stopped dropping pounds. We tried waiting until the next visit the week after and still he hadn't lost weight. He had become stagnant! Something was stopping him from losing weight. Something was blocking his metabolism. Logic told me that someone that had been having so much success for so many weeks in losing weight didn't just stop losing weight from pure chance.

In the second week that he hadn't lost weight I sat down to talk to the guy to see what had changed. At first, he didn't find anything that had changed in his weight loss routine or in his diet plan. I kept persisting until the moment he told me, "Well, last week I bought some sugar free chocolates that are low in carbohydrates". It came to my mind that NaturalSlim sells special sugar free chocolates that are low in carbohydrates for people who want to lose weight. However, the chocolates that this man bought were sweetened with a sweetener called *maltitol*, which though it doesn't contain carbohydrates, is a product derived from corn.

I suspected that perhaps this man had an intolerance to corn because I had read several books, written by doctors who are allergists, which talked about people whose bodies' rejects corn as a food. I asked him if he had noticed any intestinal gases or flatulence after ingesting the food. He told me that he had indeed. I remembered that when the body rejects any food, you don't digest it and it decomposes inside of the body, creating gases.

I asked this NaturalSlim member to do his usual routine and diet as he had learned from us but to make sure not to consume anything that could contain *maltitol* or corn. It was a miracle, the next week this man was jumping with joy because he had lost 7 pounds in that week!

In this man's case we discovered that his body was intolerant to corn and products derived from corn like *maltitol.* Since he stopped eating the chocolates and he made sure he avoided corn, the man kept on losing weight and he finally achieved his goal of losing 60 pounds from when he started.

With soy and its derived products the same thing happens. For some people, if they consume soy, they simply will not lose weight. When we first started NaturalSlim, we used a soy protein shake. We found that some people lost weight very well while others lost weight slowly or didn't lose weight at all. We started to become suspicious of soy and its "goitrogens" and we began to use whey protein (a milk protein) instead in our protein shakes. When we had the people, who didn't lose weight with the soy protein shake drink the whey protein shake, they all began to lose weight. That is how we started getting rid of all of the products that we initially offered that had soy and its derivatives.

Lastly, perhaps the most common intolerance that we have seen is the food intolerance to wheat. Wheat has a protein called "gluten" to which many people are intolerant. Wheat is the source of bread, flour and pasta. For some people eating a little bread is equivalent to not being able to lose weight. They love bread, but their bodies don't like the bread, or any foods manufactured with wheat. I am one of those cases. In my case, if I want to lose weight, I have to completely eliminate wheat from my diet. I can eat small portions of rice, potatoes and other starches. But, if I eat a bit of bread or some breaded meat, my metabolism stops, and I stop losing the body fat.

In my case, I discovered that wheat is the main food intolerance that my body has. I have seen hundreds of people with the same problem. I started buying rice crackers and potato bread in the health food stores in order to be able to enjoy toast or crackers every once in a while, without having to ingest wheat. There are numerous products in the supermarket or health food store that are "gluten-free" because there are many people that are allergic or intolerant to wheat and its protein, gluten.

I should mention that some people also have intolerances to pork meat. Pork, for some reason, isn't right for some people's bodies and it makes it very difficult for them to lose weight when they eat pork, sausage or pork rinds.

Food intolerances have to do with hereditary factors. Some of our ancestors came from Europe, others from northern countries, others from Africa, while others came from the Orient. We all carry different genes that determine which foods are acceptable and those, which are not acceptable for our bodies. Food intolerances are like allergic reactions but without obvious symptoms. They are reactions to certain foods that don't belong in our genetic heredity. In other words, they are the foods that didn't exist in the areas where our ancestors developed.

Aside from the difficulty in losing weight and the slow metabolism that corn, soy and wheat can cause, there are several warning signs that can be noted when we eat any food that our body doesn't agree with. In many cases, when we eat a food for which our body has intolerance, it creates: mucus, stomach gases, intestinal gases, water retention or constipation. Sometimes you can also feel a certain tiredness or weakness after consuming one of your offending foods.

Don't try to eliminate corn, soy or wheat from your diet. Try to DISCOVER which ones your body rejects and avoid them. I discovered that my only intolerance is to wheat. Since then I found that I could lose weight whenever I want. I just lower my intake of refined carbohydrates and eliminate wheat. My wife is intolerant to corn; she has to avoid corn in order to lose weight. Some people are intolerant to all.

The key is to start watching and paying attention. When someone eats a food that they are intolerant to it always causes certain side effects. They are subtle but noticeable body reactions, like stomach gases, intestinal gases, flatulence, mucus, as well as swelling. Swelling is caused when the body confronts a food that it considers an "enemy", the cells fill up with water and they get bigger, which causes the swelling. Swelling is water retention. After having eaten an offending food you can see how suddenly your clothes fit tighter, it takes more work to get your rings off of your fingers and your feet barely fit into your shoes. It is water retention that is caused as a reaction to the food you ate and that your body rejects.

Food intolerances don't apply to everyone. There are people that don't have any intolerance. What is important is that you know that they exist. The idea is that you can detect your body's food intolerances in your body before some food lowers your metabolism and makes you fail due to not knowing that this type of situation exists.

An additional way of finding out if your body has some sort of intolerance is by watching the cravings that you have. Oddly enough, those foods that our bodies crave the most are generally the same ones that we are intolerant to. If your body is asking for cookies, this is very likely proof that you have food intolerance to the wheat in the cookies. The foods to which our body is intolerant, is generally the same one that our body has such strong cravings for. This is also the case with sugar. Lots of people are intolerant to sugar and yet they crave it in full force.

Do the test and devote yourself to eliminating, one by one, the different foods that your body craves. If you eliminate one of the possible offending foods from your diet and during that same week you happen to lose double the usual weight that you had normally lost you will have found one of your body's intolerances. Every one of the food intolerances is like a brake for your metabolism. If you remove the food intolerances you will remove the brakes that were causing a slow metabolism. Knowledge is power!

DEFICIENT BREAKFAST

One of the worst habits of overweight people is that they don't eat an adequate breakfast. Breakfast is the most important meal of the day for anyone, but most especially for those people who want to lose weight and recover their metabolism.

When our body sleeps at night the metabolism slows down because our body enters a "repair" period. While sleeping, all of the basic functions of the body slow down and even our breathing is much slower than normal. In order to sleep it is necessary that the metabolism and production of energy slows down in the body. Experts estimate that our metabolism becomes as much as 40% slower while we are sleeping.

When you wake up in the morning your metabolism stays at a slow speed until one of two things happens: you eat food (which gives your body the signal that it should increase your metabolism) or you do exercises (which force the body to increase its production of energy and the metabolism). In other words, only two things increase the metabolism early in the morning, eating or doing exercise.

It has been found that proteins (meat, egg, cheese, etc.) and fats increase the metabolism more noticeably than carbohydrates (bread, flour, sugar, oats, etc). If one wants to "awaken" their metabolism early in the morning their breakfast should be high in proteins and low in carbohydrates.

People, who don't eat breakfast and then try to go throughout the morning with just coffee and a piece of bread, are little by little slowing down their metabolism because they simply aren't "waking" it up. The experience of helping thousands of people lose weight has shown me that a breakfast high in protein (eggs with ham and a half-slice of bread) gets a person to increase their metabolism and gives him a chance at losing weight. If the morning protein is in the form of a whey protein shake, then the results will be even better.

There is a popular saying that expresses what our food intake should be like. The saying goes "we should eat breakfast like a king, eat lunch like a prince, and eat dinner like a beggar". This saying is true. The most important meal of the day is breakfast. It is called "breakfast" because it is the moment that you "break the fast" of the long hours in which your body was sleeping and repairing itself. The longest period in which our body is without food is during the hours in which we are sleeping.

The lightest meal of the day should be dinner. Foods are made of condensed energy. Eating too heartily at night forces an entrance of energy (food) to the body and going to sleep lowers your energy use, which forces a "storage mode" (fat). It is an aspect of pure logic; dinner should be like a beggar, not like a king.

In my case, I had to change my habits to be able to overcome obesity. My habit when I was obese was that I didn't eat breakfast. I just drank a cup of coffee early in the morning and went to work. For lunch I ate "whatever there was" without thinking about it much. Dinner was always the biggest meal of the day. I always ate dinners that were high in refined carbohydrates (rice, bread, potato, etc.) along with a sweet dessert. After dinner I felt so tired and sleepy that I would generally fall asleep while watching television. It was the equivalent of filling the tanks of an airplane with high octane gasoline and later turning off all the airplane's engines so that the energy is conserved and stored. Eating too heartily at night and going to sleep is a sure way to cause weight problems or obesity.

If you want to strengthen your metabolism, it is necessary to begin your day with eating a breakfast high in proteins that is good enough for a king. Later, continue on to a lunch that has a good combination of proteins and unrefined carbohydrates (vegetables, salads). Make sure to consume very little refined carbohydrates (rice, flour, bread, sugar, etc.). Finally, end the day with a light dinner to prepare your body for its period of sleep and restoration. In conclusion, it is necessary to understand the way in which the human body functions and establish a lifestyle that includes eating food that contributes to your metabolism.

CANDIDA ALBICANS YEAST, "THE SILENT EPIDEMIC"

In my company, NaturalSlim, more than hundreds of thousands of people have been helped in losing weight and recovering their metabolism. In the process of working with so many people that wanted to lose weight, we learned a lot. We had the opportunity of discovering various factors that are of true importance for anyone that wants to recover their metabolism and leave behind being overweight or obese once and for all.

The topic of the *candida albicans*[17] yeast is vital information. It is something so important to know about that when we discovered that this yeast lowers the metabolism of the body, we began to use a natural yeast-cleansing program in NaturalSlim and our success rate nearly doubled. In starting to treat the yeast infections of our NaturalSlim system members, we succeeded in helping more people lose weight, even those who had failed in all of their previous efforts. We saw some incredible things, like the case of a woman who managed to go from a size 22 down to a size 6 after doing the yeast cleansing; it was amazing! We had discovered the solution to one of the worst causes of a "slow metabolism" and this, more than anything else, guaranteed our success.

---

[17] *Candida albicans*: yeast that lives in all human bodies. There are different varieties of yeasts. The variety called "albicans" is the most prevalent in the bodies of people who are diabetics, have weight problems, or who are obese. "Albicans" means "white". In fact, at times this yeast can be found as white spots on newborn babies' tongues whose mothers were infected with the *candida albicans* yeast.

Candida albicans is one of the many organisms that live inside the human body. Different organisms exist most especially in the intestinal area, called the "gut flora", and the vaginal area (in the case of women) called "the "vaginal flora". Within these organisms there are different classes of bacteria, various types of yeasts, viruses and certain types of parasites. We don't necessarily like to think of these types of things, but the truth is, that various types of organisms like these survive inside of our body.

All humans are born with the candida yeast as part of their intestinal and vaginal flora. It is a natural organism in all humans. It is for this same reason that traditional medicine hasn't placed much importance on the subject. However, since the 1980's various prominent allergists and specialists in infectious organisms have given the voice of alert about the growing infections of the candida yeast.

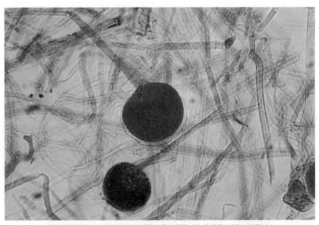

CANDIDA ALBICANS YEAST CLOSE UP VIEW

Dr. William G. Crook, an allergist, with his book, *"Yeast Connection Handbook"*, is possibly the main exponent of what some have called "the silent epidemic of the *candida albicans* yeast". When this yeast has overgrown in the body, it causes what is called a "systemic infection". It is at this point that the candida yeast is transported through the blood and it invades other organs in the body creating serious health and metabolism problems. People with systemic infections from this yeast always have a "slow metabolism" and can't lose weight under any diet or exercise plan. If they do lose weight, they do it at such a slow rate that they generally get discouraged.

A researcher of this subject found that the *candida albicans* yeast produces 78 different toxins inside the body and this creates a toxic and acidic environment inside the body, which basically turns off the metabolism. Having a very developed candida colony or an "overgrowth" of this yeast in the body is one of the main reasons why some people have a "slow metabolism". As long as they have this yeast infection in their body, no effort they make to lose weight will work for them. The body of a person who has an "overgrowth" of the candida yeast is full of toxins produced by the yeast.

Yeasts like *candida albicans* create "mycotoxins[18]". This is a well-known fact by experts in toxic substances. For example, there are yeasts that produce a poisonous toxin called "aflatoxin" that has been proven to be highly carcinogenic (causes cancer) and has been used as a biological war weapon by some countries. In some cases, the yeast has produced mycotoxins that have poisoned livestock food and have led to many deaths of the animals that livestock owners breed. Farm animals often die or suffer from mycotoxin poisoning. Mycotoxins are powerful poisons that have the ability of paralyzing the respiratory and nervous systems of its victims.

In my experience, nothing produces an increase of the metabolism and allows more noticeable weight loss like doing a program of a candida yeast body cleansing.

---

[18] Mycotoxins – toxins produced by an organism of the fungi kingdom, which includes mushrooms, molds and yeasts. Mycotoxins vary greatly in their severity. Some mycotoxins are lethal, some cause identifiable diseases or health problems, some weaken the immune system without producing symptoms specific to that toxin and some act as allergens or irritants.

There are laboratory tests to detect if your *candida albicans* yeast infection is severe, but the tests that measure the various toxin levels that produce this yeast in the blood cost more than $300 and really are not available in the majority of laboratories. The best way to find out if this yeast infects your body is to use a list of "indicators" that was developed by Dr. William Cook for his patients. Perhaps the clearest signs that you have a severe infection of *candida albicans* in your body are itching on your skin (mainly at night or after showering); you often have stomach or intestinal gases after eating, having sinusitis or suffering from migraines. The complete list of the symptoms of *candida albicans* is the following:

- Acne
- Allergies in humid environments
- Allergies to some foods
- Allergies to certain metal jewelry
- Continuously tired
- Urinary tract infections (cystitis)
- Constant or frequent diarrhea
- Pain or vaginal burning while having sex
- Headaches or migraines
- Severe menstrual pain—PMS
- Muscular pain
- Constipation
- Fatigue or weakness
- Vaginal itching or discharge
- Coldness in extremities (hands or feet)
- Excessive stomach or intestinal gases
- Ear infections
- Urinary tract infections
- Irregularity or troubles with menstruation
- Irritability or depression
- Itchy skin (especially at night or after showering)
- Digestive gas problems
- Excessive dryness of the skin
- A "taste of metal" in the mouth

- Rash or spots on skin after sunbathing
- Sensitivity to solar light, teary eyes
- Sensitivity to odors from cigarettes, perfumes or chemicals
- Sinusitis

The more of these symptoms you have in your body the more severe will be the infection of the candida yeast. I recognize that this list of symptoms is lengthy, and a person can begin to justify their symptoms based on other sicknesses or hereditary factors that their body has. The reality is that when a person does a candida yeast body cleansing, the majority, if not all of these symptoms disappear completely. This is true in all cases, especially in the cases of people that suffer from sinusitis or migraines. Throughout the years, we have observed how case after case, the sinusitis and migraines simply disappeared after having cleaned the body of this yeast using natural fungicides (substances that kill funguses or yeasts).

Our interest always has been in helping people recover their metabolism and lose weight. The almost miraculous recoveries from conditions like sinusitis or migraines are just the added benefits of what we do to help them recover the metabolism. It's just that we couldn't help but notice that after a natural candida yeast cleansing program people are finally able to lose weight much faster and the cleanse also eliminates the majority of the symptoms that this yeast causes.

Doctors refer to the severe *candida albicans* yeast infection condition as "candidiasis", but they generally only associate it with cancer patients in their terminal state and with patients that have Acquired Immunodeficiency Syndrome (AIDS). The traditional medical point of view is that since we all have the *candida albicans* yeast it couldn't be a very serious problem unless the person has a very weak immune system. We can't blame doctors for the low ability to observe their patient's symptoms in the case of the candida yeast as they only receive limited information about this subject in medical school.

In fact, some of the most difficult members to help on the NaturalSlim system have been people in the medical profession. When we have told some of them the importance of reducing the body's colony of the *candida albicans* yeast, so that they can successfully lose weight quickly, some of them have responded with resistance to the subject. However, when these doctors followed our recommendations and did do a natural yeast-cleansing program, all of them experienced amazing results that turned them into firm believers of the importance of reducing the candida yeast in the body, to be able to increase the metabolism and lose weight. These days, there have been many doctors in our weight loss system that have verified, by their own personal experience, that reducing the *candida albicans* yeast infection is indeed vital if one wants to be successful in losing weight and recovering the metabolism.

Traditional medicine uses medicines like Diflucan, Nystatin, Mycostatin, Nizerol and Sporanox, along with other fungicides to try and kill the *candida albicans* yeast. However, even though these medications can help in the cases of people with cancer or AIDS, they are labeled with strong warnings due to the toxic effects and permanent liver damage that they can cause. The types of chemical substances that these medications contain are toxic not only to the *candida albicans* yeast but also to many of the other cells in the body. That's why we developed a natural candida yeast-cleansing program, to have a way of reducing the yeast colony in the body and to get the person to recover their metabolism and lose weight. Many of the people that seek help from the NaturalSlim system are people that have "tried everything" without good results. We know from experience that if you don't succeed in reducing the infection of the *candida albicans* yeast in your body, you will not lose weight effectively.

Reducing a severe infection of this yeast is not an easy task. When we attack the yeast with natural fungicides, like oregano, the reactions can be really unpleasant (headaches, diarrhea, muscular pain, etc.). We have had to learn to increase the dose of the natural fungicides "little by little". On the other hand, to be successful, you can't use common oregano oil like what they sell in natural health food stores. The regular oregano oil reduces the infection of *candida albicans* only in the intestine and this is not good enough, given that the candida infection generally is spread throughout the entire body. Throughout the years and hundreds of tests and trials, we succeeded in finding a natural oregano oil supplement that is emulsified. An emulsion is a mixture of two generally unblendable substances like water and oil. The active yeast-killing ingredient in oregano is an oily substance called *carvacol*. Oils don't mix well with water and our blood is primarily composed of water. This oregano oil supplement has the advantage of being emulsified and thus mixes well and travels well in the blood and kills the yeast in all of the parts of the body where it could be invading it.

The *candida albicans* yeast colony in the body can never be eliminated 100% since this yeast is a natural inhabitant of the body. The strategy that is used is reducing the yeast colony to the point in which it stops being a problem for the metabolism. If a yeast infection is reduced in size, say from 100% to 20%, we will have had success and the person will be rewarded for their efforts by losing weight. They will also experience an obvious improvement in their general state of health.

A main discovery has been that this yeast, that normally only inhabits a small part of the intestinal and vaginal flora, can grow to the point of occupying the majority of the internal flora of the body, turning into an aggressive parasite that invades all parts of the body. The infection of the *candida albicans* yeast is possibly one of the main and less well-known causes of the epidemic of weight problems and obesity that affect numerous countries in the world. This has not happened by pure chance. There are factors that have allowed this yeast, which normally doesn't affect us, to reproduce at such a fast rate and has turned it into a parasite that leaves the intestine and vaginal area and invades the rest of the body, causing a systemic (body wide) infection that affects all of the body's organs from the brain to the liver.

In order to resolve the problems that the candida yeast causes for the metabolism and health, it is vital to educate the infected person about the characteristics of his or her internal enemy, *candida albicans*. If one wants to overcome an enemy it is important to know the enemy's characteristics and weak points. Part of the strategy is to educate the person so that they don't unknowingly contribute to creating a suitable environment for the growth of this yeast and so that they don't in a short time go back to having a new "overgrowth" that lowers their metabolism. The education includes making the person understand which factors are the ones that promote the growth of this yeast inside their body. The factors that contribute to the "overgrowth" of the candida yeast are:

EXCESS OF REFINED CARBOHYDRATES:
Refined carbohydrates (sugar, candy, bread, rice, etc.) produce an excess of glucose in the blood and this excess of glucose feeds the raging appetite of the candida yeast and makes it grow excessively. It's like putting fertilizer on a weed. When someone maintains high levels of glucose in their body due to their diet high in refined carbohydrates or sweet carbohydrates, the yeast feeds off of it voraciously, which makes it grow and reproduce at an accelerated rate. Glucose is the main food for all of the cells in our body. It is also the main food for the *candida albicans* yeast. Someone who is accustomed to eating a lot of sweet foods will see their metabolism lower year after year until it turns into a "slow metabolism".

TAKING ANTIBIOTICS:
Antibiotics get rid of the bacteria that cause infections in the body, but they also get rid of the "good bacteria" that live in the intestine and vaginal area that are natural enemies of the *candida albicans* yeast. When the intestinal and vaginal flora die due to the dose of antibiotics, the yeast is left without competition and opposition and it invades the rest of the body quickly. When someone finds himself or herself obligated to take antibiotics, they should make sure to also take a supplement to replace the intestinal bacteria with "friendly bacteria". The "friendly bacteria" have names like *acidophilus, bulgaricus* and *bifidus*. In all-natural food stores, they

offer supplements that contain these types of beneficial bacteria, which replace the lost "friendly bacteria" that the antibiotic medicine killed and that way your body isn't missing the intestinal and vaginal friendly bacteria that protect you from the candida yeast.

TAKING ESTROGEN (FEMALE HORMONES):
Contraceptive pills, estrogen patches and medications for menopause speed up the growth of this yeast and cause an "overgrowth". Many women lose their beautiful figure after using contraceptive pills or contraceptive patches for just a few months. Estrogen, of course, is a hormone that accumulates fat and makes you fat, but also has the effect of being a "growth factor" for the *candida albicans* yeast. In other words, it allows this yeast to grow quicker.

TAKING CORTISONE:
This medication, cortisone, which is used to lower inflammation in the body, also lowers the immune system and causes the *candida albicans* yeast to grow increasingly faster, which then lowers the metabolism. For example, people who suffer from asthma use an inhaler with a medication derived from cortisone. In addition, many of these people not only suffer from asthma, but they also start to have weight and obesity problems.

DRINKING ALCOHOLIC BEVERAGES:
When someone has a systemic infection of the candida yeast they should avoid drinking alcoholic beverages (wine, beer, whiskey, rum, etc.) since this yeast lives on alcohol much easier than sugar.

THYROID GLAND PROBLEMS:
The thyroid gland and its related systems control the body's metabolism, temperature and immune system. It is a fact that people with hypothyroidism suffer from frequent colds and infections because their immune system is low. People that have deficient thyroid gland systems tend to have strong infections of this candida yeast. This happens because their immunological systems

are not protecting them from the yeast with the normal efficiency of an agile immune system.

It is vital to know the factors that make the *candida albicans* yeast grow inside your body. If someone intends on lowering their level of infection of the candida yeast but doesn't take into consideration these factors that contribute to create a favorable environment for the yeast, then not much time will pass before their metabolism is lowered by a new increase of the infection with this yeast. The idea is to reduce the infection in order to recover the metabolism and change your "lifestyle" to see that this yeast doesn't come back with equal or greater force. It's about changing your habits so that you don't keep feeding and catering to this parasitic organism, *candida albicans*.

Diabetics, as a result of their diabetic condition, are extremely infected with the *candida albicans* yeast. Diabetes, by definition, is a condition in which glucose levels are abnormally high. It could be said that the body of a diabetic is like a paradise for yeasts like *candida albicans* because of its constant high abundance of glucose.

This topic about the infections of the *candida albicans* yeast has, quite possibly, been the most controversial topic that I have run into, in my search for the reasons for the so-called "slow metabolism". Oddly enough, it is also the topic that has produced the best results for those thousands of people that had already lost their hope of being able to lose weight. Still, after many years, I can't help but be amazed by the positive results that lowering the *candida albicans* yeast infection can do for your body. After a *candida albicans* yeast cleansing program, I've seen the weight loss and health recovery of people that before didn't have hope of ever achieving it.

There is an incalculable satisfaction in finding the cause and solution to a health and metabolism problem like this infection with the *candida albicans* yeast.

DIABETES AND HYPOGLYCEMIA

Diabetes, as much as hypoglycemia[19], has a direct relation with a deficient metabolism.

There are two types of diabetes. Type-II diabetes is the most common, as approximately 90% of diabetics have type II. It is a condition of diabetes that starts when the person is an adult. Diabetes type I is hereditary diabetes, which is much less common, where the person is born with a pancreas that simply doesn't produce any *insulin*. That's why the type I diabetic has to inject themselves with *insulin* 3 or 4 times a day for their entire life.

Diabetes is a condition in which the body maintains glucose levels (blood sugar) that are too high and this in turn affects the health and metabolism of the person. Glucose levels are measured in milligrams per deciliter[20] (mg/dl). It is a measurement that laboratories use to find out if a person is suffering from diabetes. Normal levels are from 75 to 125 mg/dl depending on what and when the person ate. Diabetics maintain glucose levels of above 130 mg/dl and in some cases, it can get up to 500 mg/dl and the person goes unconscious because of the excess of glucose.

The American Diabetes Association estimated a few years ago that there were about 14 million diabetics in the United States or about 6.2% of the population that suffers from this condition. The statistics are clear, diabetes is growing at a fast rate and medical and health authorities in the country really don't know what to do to stop this condition.

---

[19] Hypoglycemia - is a medical term referring to a state produced by a lower than normal level of glucose (sugar) in the blood.

[20] Deciliter – a measure of liquid volume equal to a liter divided in 10 parts.

No part of the population is as sick as diabetics. Diabetics are the part of the population that suffers from the most heart attacks, loss of vision and many times have to use dialysis treatments (mechanized system to clean the blood) when their kidneys fail completely. What's more, at least 85% of diabetics are overweight or obese. What's worse is that diabetic males in many cases become sexually impotent. It is clear; diabetics really are the least healthy people in our population.

Scientists constantly fill the pages of newspapers with their "discoveries" of supposed diabetic genes and try to blame it on heredity factors. According to their theories, the blame always seems to be on the human body; it is in some way defective and therefore is diabetic. The given impression is that the person is a poor "victim" and that the person has nothing to do with the fact that they are diabetic.

Well, my experience with diabetics, in the process of helping them lose weight and recover their metabolisms, has been very enlightening. I've worked with more than 2,000 diabetic people and have seen amazing results, not only in successfully losing weight, but also in seeing how they have been able to control their diabetes.

In order to help the diabetics, the only information that was useful to me throughout the years was the information published by Dr. Richard Bernstein in his book, *"Diabetes Solution"*. I would recommend that every diabetic read this book, so that once and for all they can understand their condition and be able to control it. It terrifies me to think about some of the advice that "experts" in nutrition have been giving their diabetic patients. Some recommendations like "have snacks every 2-3 hours so that your blood sugar stay's stable."

My experience is that diabetes is simply an <u>inability of the body to process refined carbohydrates</u>. In other words, a diabetic's body has severe problems when it is fed foods like bread, flour, candy, chocolate, rice, potato, fruit, etc. If the diabetic eats sweet carbohydrates like, raisins, banana, or mangos, they will also have problems. If they eat natural carbohydrates (vegetables, salads) they don't have any problems. Refined carbohydrates are deadly for diabetics.

I am used to seeing people with diabetes adjust their diet to one that is low in refined carbohydrates and immediately they begin losing weight and controlling their diabetes. So, a typical Mediterranean diet, like meat, cheese and salads for a diabetic is perfect. I've seen diabetics who would inject themselves with 60 units of insulin daily, get to the point where they don't have to use insulin anymore and they can control their blood sugar with only a medication to control their glucose. By lowering their intake of refined carbohydrates, their blood sugar levels started to normalize. Due to this, their doctors found themselves forced to reduce their medication dosage. I've seen them come in with large pieces of dead, black skin on their feet and I've also seen how this skin is regenerated and goes back to a pinkish, healthy color when they control their refined carbohydrates.

One of the most interesting experiences that I've had was with a diabetic doctor that sought out our help at NaturalSlim. This doctor is one of the most well-organized people I have ever met. He measured his glucose level several times a day and kept a detailed agenda noting everything that he ate and what affect it had on his glucose. He started to lose weight noticeably and had to go down to taking less than half of his medications in order to control his glucose. When he broke his diet and gave in to some bread or refined carbohydrates he also noted and observed that his glucose rose once more to dangerous levels. In the end, the doctor discovered the same as I had, that diabetes is completely controllable if you can control your consumption of refined carbohydrates.

In my experience, no one sees a more noticeable improvement than diabetics, when they control their consumption of refined carbohydrates. Whether a type I or type II diabetic, the key is lowering the intake of refined carbohydrates to a minimum. Precisely so, Dr. Richard Bernstein's recommendation in his book is to substantially reduce the consumption of refined carbohydrates. He is right; I have experienced it with thousands of diabetics. When the intake of refined carbohydrates is decreased, all cases of diabetes are controlled, blood pressure goes down, triglycerides are lower and bad cholesterol (LDL) is also reduced. I've never been able to understand why something so simple is not explained to diabetics. Controlling diabetes is completely based on controlling the consumption of refined carbohydrates (bread, flour, candy, chocolates, rice, potatoes, grits, etc.) At times, I have thought that there are financially motivated "vested interests", that don't want diabetes to be controlled, so that they can keep on earning a bunch of money from the sales of medications and treatments that they make for diabetics. The solution is as simple as controlling your refined carbohydrates. However, they trick diabetics with an extensive variety of "sugar-free" products that, in reality, are high in refined carbohydrates (wheat flour, honey, molasses, etc.)

I have attended the Diabetes Association trade shows and have seen how they recommend "sugar-free" candy products to diabetics without explaining to them that ALL carbohydrates turn into sugar (glucose) when they enter the digestive system. Under this false idea that all "sugar-free" products don't affect them, they sell cookies, cakes and candies that, within minutes of eating them, have made the glucose levels of the body go out of control. Ignorance is truly dangerous. Ignorance kills.

Diabetes is characterized by having glucose levels that are too high and hypoglycemia is characterized by having glucose levels that are too low. They seem like they are opposite conditions, but they are not. They are related, and you should know that hypoglycemia would eventually turn into diabetes if you don't change your diet and lifestyle.

In reality, hypoglycemia or "low blood sugar", is only intolerance to refined carbohydrates. Hypoglycemia is the beginning of a problem where the body starts giving off an alarm that it doesn't want refined carbohydrates. Diabetes is the final stage of the problem that has already turned into an inability to utilize refined carbohydrates. We could say that hypoglycemia is comparable to a "protest" or "work strike" and diabetes represents a failed company that closed its operations because it couldn't keep going.

People who are suffering from hypoglycemia are in a favorable position because they can avoid diabetes. But in order to do it, they have to stop forcing their body to accept the refined carbohydrates that it doesn't want.

The sequence of a hypoglycemic person (low blood sugar) is like this: the person stuffs themselves with refined carbohydrates or sweet carbohydrates that their body doesn't tolerate very well. The refined carbohydrates turn into an excess of glucose and their body reacts by producing too much insulin with the purpose of lowering the increase of glucose in their blood. The production of insulin of a hypoglycemic person is exaggerated and produces too much insulin in order to counteract the excess glucose which then causes the "low blood sugar" that we call hypoglycemia. If the person hadn't abused the refined carbohydrates in the first place, the excess insulin never would have been produced to cause the "low blood sugar" that is called hypoglycemia. In the end, a person that wants to stop being hypoglycemic only has to stop eating an excess of refined carbohydrates and they will see their hypoglycemia disappear forever.

There is something about explanations that are too simple. People tend to think that the solution to a problem like hypoglycemia should always be some extremely complex factor. If the solution seems too simple, many times we can't accept it. However, the solution to hypoglycemia is simple: controlling refined carbohydrates. This hypoglycemia issue is worth solving because if you are hypoglycemic and don't do anything about it, you will end up with diabetes.

Even more, when your metabolism is made slow, your body accumulates lots of fat. Fat creates two compounds, *"resistin" and "tumor necrosis factor-alpha"; these* interfere with insulin and makes the insulin ineffective. The excess body fat of a diabetic makes it so that their insulin can't extract glucose from their blood effectively and a so-called "insulin resistance" starts, where the body of the diabetic resists the effects of its own insulin and the glucose level continues rising in the blood. Finally, diabetes is aggravated, following the increase of fat in the body.

The good news is that diabetes can be controlled and hypoglycemia can be completely eliminated if you control your consumption of refined carbohydrates.

FEMALE HORMONES

Women's bodies are more complex than men's due to their hormonal system. It is a well-known fact that men lose weight easily, while women experience much more difficulty in losing weight. This is due to the following reasons:

- Men have more muscle and therefore use more energy and "burn" fat easier.

- Men produce the male hormone *testosterone,* which is a muscle constructing and fat burner hormone.

- Women produce the hormone *estrogen*, which is a hormone that accumulates fat in the body.

- Women tend to have higher emotional stress levels than men and therefore produce higher levels of the stress hormone *cortisol*, which is a hormone that accumulates fat in the abdomen and hips

It is due to these factors that women always lose weight slower than men. One of the reasons, the excess of the hormone *estrogen*, has to do with a condition that many women, especially overweight ones, suffer from. The condition is called "estrogen predominance".

This hormone, *estrogen*, in reality is a group of various substances that are vital to a woman's body. Without *estrogen,* pregnancy couldn't exist, nor would they have menstruation, breasts or soft skin.

Estrogen is a hormone that a woman's body balances with another hormone that is produced during ovulation called *progesterone. Progesterone* is a hormone that reflects its name very well because it allows "gestation" or becoming pregnant. Women's bodies depend on a certain hormonal balance between these two hormones, *estrogen* and *progesterone.*

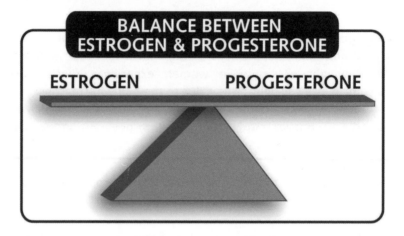

Just about everyone knows that estrogen is produced in the ovaries of a woman. But few know that the body's fat also produces *estrogen* with the help of an enzyme called *aromatase.* Fat produces *estrogen* and that's why obese men develop breasts and start to have more feminine characteristics, even to the point where their tone of voice changes in pitch.

In his book, *"What Your Doctor May Not Tell You About Menopause",* Dr. John Lee explains the problem of "estrogen predomination" in women. It is a condition where the body of an overweight woman keeps producing *estrogen* from her fat even if her ovaries don't work anymore. When the *estrogen* isn't being balanced in the body by the *progesterone* hormone, which is only produced during ovulation, it creates an "estrogen predominance" that doesn't allow the woman to lose weight. A "predomination" means that the *estrogen* dominates the body internally because the *progesterone* isn't there to oppose it. This creates a situation that makes it very difficult for women to lose weight because the excess *estrogen* accumulates fat and makes you gain weight and, at the same time, doesn't allow fat loss.

The problem is that the *estrogen* hormone accumulates fat and makes you gain weight. This has been a well-known fact for many years; you might have seen in the news, that, some years ago the pig and hen breeders tried to make their animals gain weight by supplementing their diet with *estrogen* to make them fatter. This was publicized on the front pages of newspapers around the country as a scandal and as a result, many people decided not to continue consuming chicken meat. As far as I know, this practice isn't continued today, but many people are still upset about the attempted manipulation in using *estrogen* to make the animals gain weight. They still refuse to consume chicken due to fear that it contains *estrogen*.

When a woman suffers from an "estrogen predomination" she can experience the following symptoms:

- Accumulation of fat in the hips and abdomen
- Re-occurring yeast infections
- Autoimmune conditions like: Lupus, Multiple Sclerosis and Fibromyalgia
- Difficulty losing weight or losing weight very slowly
- Difficulty becoming pregnant
- Water retention (edema)
- Lack of energy or constantly tired
- History of breast or uterine cancer
- History of fibroids, adenomas or vaginal polyps
- History of having miscarriages
- Painful menstruation or cramps
- Osteoporosis (loss of bone density)
- Facial hair
- Loss of sexual interest or appetite
- Excessive menstrual bleeding

- Breast tenderness
- Sleeping too lightly or sleeping difficulties

"Estrogen predomination" keeps the metabolism low and makes it very difficult for the woman suffering from this condition to lose weight.

Estrogen is a growth promoting agent for cancerous cells, which is why having "estrogen predominance", puts a woman at a high risk for breast and uterine cancer.

When a woman starts getting a lot of facial hair, it is generally a result of the "estrogen predominance" that makes the body produce more masculine hormones (androgens) to counteract the *estrogen*. The body will do its best to try and balance out the "estrogen predominance" by producing more masculine hormones if it can't produce the *progesterone* it needs. This increases facial and body hair.

The solution for women is to use a natural *progesterone* cream. This natural hormone is applied to the skin and counteracts the harmful effects of the "estrogen predominance", successfully balancing the hormonal system. The natural *progesterone* has a calming and antidepressant effect. Also, it helps women have deeper, sounder sleep.

You use the natural *progesterone* cream for just 21 days out of the month so that your body doesn't become accustomed to it and stops reacting properly to it. Women that still have periods should start using it on the first day of their period and use it for 21 days. On the 21st day stop using it and give yourself a rest and then go back to using it again when your next cycle starts.

If a woman no longer has a period (menopause), she uses it for 21 days, but starts on the 1st day of every month until the 21st. The idea is to create a *progesterone* supplementation cycle as if it were the body itself that would still be producing the *progesterone* through ovulation.

You can get this cream at most natural product stores or you can get it through the Internet. For women that have experienced a great deal of difficulty in losing weight and especially those that have gained a lot of weight in their hips and abdomen (caused by *estrogen*), the natural *progesterone* cream can be an excellent help.

Along with all of these benefits, natural *progesterone* also has an anti-aging effect on the body. Women who use natural *progesterone* have nicer skin. The only additional comment from women who use it is that it causes an increase of libido (sexual appetite). Notice that natural *progesterone* has always been used to help women that suffer from sexual frigidity. It is a hormone that promotes "gestation" (pregnancy) and therefore increases sexual interest. Many husbands know about the libido enhancing properties of this hormone and suggest that their partner use the natural *progesterone* cream regularly every month.

Natural *progesterone* also has an effect of detaining bone loss or even helping to recover bone that has been lost due to a condition called osteoporosis[21]. This is something that can be proven 3 months after having begun to use the cream by doing a bone density exam and comparing it to an exam done before using natural *progesterone.*

I recommended that you buy and read the book by Dr. John Lee on this topic. Don't assume that your own doctor knows about this topic, since our doctors depend almost entirely on the scientific information that is provided to them on a continuing basis by the

---

[21] Osteoporosis - is a disease of bone leading to an increased risk of fracture. In osteoporosis the bone mineral density is reduced. Osteoporosis is most common in women after the menopause but may develop in men and premenopausal women in the presence of particular hormonal disorders.

pharmaceutical companies. For pharmaceutical companies, natural *progesterone* isn't good business because of the fact that it is natural and can't be protected with a patent, so you can't make much money off of it. If your doctor isn't familiar with the subject, he or she will tell you not to use any hormones, whether they are natural or not, and this is understandable since they have been attacked with frivolous and, in many cases, unjust lawsuits for malpractice. In my experience, if the doctor isn't familiar with the subject, he or she will recommend that you don't do anything about it so that they can protect themselves from being legally responsible for their uninformed advice. The standard answer is always "no" or "don't use" if they are uninformed about the subject. This is an understandable attitude that doctors have, since many of them are being sued unjustly for malpractice. So, if the doctor doesn't know about the subject of *progesterone* he or she will surely tell a woman not to use it.

If you want to know more about this subject, inform and educate yourself so that you can have your own opinions about it. It is your body and thus it is your responsibility to know.

I can tell you that if your weight or obesity problem is concentrated in lower parts of your body (hips and abdomen) and you are feeling various symptoms like those described for "estrogen predominance", you could experience a miracle in starting to use the natural *progesterone* cream. When the "estrogen predominance" is very strong, the use of the natural *progesterone* cream causes an amazing increase in the metabolism and helps achieve the hormonal balance that your body needs to stay at its optimum state.

ANTIDEPRESSANTS AND MEDICATIONS THAT MAKE YOU GAIN WEIGHT

Antidepressant medications, all of them, make you gain weight. Generally, the manufacturer assumes its responsibility and says it on the "warning" page that comes with these medications. My experience has been that very few things lower the metabolism more than antidepressant medications (*Zoloft, Paxil, Prozac* and others). All of them make you gain weight!

I've seen hundreds of people, mostly women, who start using an antidepressant and they start to gain weight much faster. Also, the efforts that they make to help increase their metabolism produce very little results. I know that this is true because, in the cases where someone got to the point where they could stop using anti-depressant medication, they automatically started to lose weight.

Over the years I've learned about using natural supplements that have an antidepressant effect like the amino acid L-Tyrosine, vitamin B-1 (thiamine). There is also a natural Russian herb called *rhodiola rosea* that some American psychiatrists have begun using in their private practices for their patients with depression.

When we are interested in fighting a "slow metabolism" we have to learn to distinguish which are the medications that lower our metabolism, and antidepressants definitely make you gain weight. Your psychiatrist can insist that these are just "stories" but if you look at your waist line you will see that what I am telling you is true. Your clothes don't lie!

Another group of medications that lower the metabolism and make you gain weight are diuretic medications that are used to lower your blood pressure. It turns out that everything that increases water in your body tends to increase the metabolism and everything that lowers the water level of your body decreases it. Diuretics work by lowering water levels in the body to lower the pressure. Numerous times I've seen how a person starts having a much slower metabolism after starting to take diuretic medications.

The best way to lower your blood pressure is to lose weight. There is a direct relation between being overweight and having high blood pressure. Losing weight almost always gets your blood pressure to go back down to normal. Your body fat produces a substance called *"angiotensinogen"*, which is associated to high blood pressure. The more fat there is in your body, the more tendencies there will be for you to have high blood pressure. If you lower your body fat, your blood pressure lowers and normalizes, unless you have one of those very rare cases of high blood pressure caused by stress or emotions. Losing weight and lowering your body fat are the real solutions.

If you currently use a diuretic medicine to lower your blood pressure, don't make the mistake of stopping its use until you have lost weight and your blood pressure has gone back to normal. These medications can't be stopped or reduced without the help of your doctor.

Other medications that make you gain weight are those that are used for inflammations in your body. For example, the inhalers that asthmatics use, cortisone injections for back inflammations or cortisone tablets (Prednisone an others) for other inflammatory conditions like arthritis. These are medications chemically related to cortisone. Cortisone is a hormone that is identical to the *cortisol* that our body produces in the adrenal glands. It is called "cortisone" when it is produced by the pharmaceutical industry and *"cortisol"* when our body produces it, but they are basically the same hormone.

All in all, what you need to know is that there are medications that decrease your metabolism. Naturally, medications can be necessary depending on the condition. But it is also true that when a person increases their metabolism and loses weight, a majority of their health problems improve or disappear completely. I've seen hundreds of cases of people that have lost weight and get to the point where their doctor discontinued the medications they took for their condition. The human body has an apparently infinite ability to recuperate from any condition when we give it the help it needs to do so.

SEDENTARY LIFESTYLE

Our current lifestyle includes a large variety of technological advances that do not require our physical activity. Nowadays, we are surrounded by cell phones, microwaves, televisions, computers, vacuum cleaners and numerous other kinds of equipment that require very little physical effort to operate.

The present tendency is to move our bodies less and use more of our mind and senses. We are often sports spectators as opposed to actually playing sports ourselves. The daily "rush" seems to leave little time for exercising, walking, swimming or any other type of body movement. In general, we even use our cars to drive to the next corner to get some necessity when we could have walked a little. On the other hand, we sometimes fear for our security and "walking to the corner store" may not be the best option depending on the neighborhood.

Even children today spend a good part of their time and energy playing electronic games, when years ago they played and sweated with enthusiasm. Watching television has turned into a main activity as much for children as it has for adults. We live lives of little or no physical activity; a sedentary life.

It has been proven that physical activity increases the metabolism and a sedentary life decreases it. The human body is a living organism that learns and adapts to existing conditions. When we stop using our muscles they become flaccid. When we use them, they grow and strengthen. Our body adapts to our lifestyle.

Now, even though the former is true, I'm not going to ask you to start doing exercises if you feel your metabolism is very slow. It's not the time to criticize you because of your lack of desire to exercise your body.

The years that I've spent helping people with "slow metabolism" have taught me to observe what works and what doesn't work. The fact that you have a slow metabolism, proven by your difficulties in losing weight, does not mean that it is time to start doing exercise or buying a membership to a gym. Exercise is a great help and is vital in being able to recover the maximum possible of your metabolism, but everything in life has its appropriate time and exercise is not an exception to this rule.

Logic tells us that to be able to do exercise, a person needs to expend energy. But people with slow metabolism have very little energy! That's exactly what having a "slow metabolism" means, it is having too little energy because your metabolism is what produces the body's energy. People that suffer from slow metabolism are always tired and feel weak. It is illogical to ask a weak and tired person to spend whatever little available energy they have to go to the gym and exercise. It's like trying to go on a spending spree with no money available in your checking account. In order to spend some energy in exercise you must first have it available.

When a person with slow metabolism that is also overweight or obese gets into an exercise routine, they put themselves at risk of failing in their attempt because it is forcing their body to a point that is further than the limit of their capacity. 70 % of people with new gym memberships stop going within just a few weeks of having started and paid their annual membership fee. They are weak, tired people that really don't have the necessary energy to do exercise for very long without collapsing from exhaustion. They are people that have a slow metabolism.

The solution to this problem is to apply the CORRECT SEQUENCE. In life, things have a sequence; they have an order. The correct sequence of actions is: improve your nutrition and metabolism to obtain more energy and then use this new energy in an exercise routine that increases your metabolism even more. In other words, it is depositing enough money in your checking account so that later you can go write checks to spend the money. Using checks without having available funds in your bank account leads to "bounced checks". In the same way, doing exercise without first having enough energy makes us fail in the attempt due to the lack of energy to continue.

Within a few days of having incorporated a diet plan that includes more proteins (meat, cheese, eggs) and less refined carbohydrates (bread, flour, rice, potatoes, sweets) you will feel a considerable increase of energy. Also, by drinking more water and taking a high potency vitamin and mineral supplements you will create a surplus of body energy that you can then use to start doing light exercises which will increase your metabolism even more. If someone starts eating a good breakfast and then adds to it the organic coconut oil supplement, not only will they have more energy to put into exercise, they will also feel the desire to move their body. The additional energy that a proper diet creates makes people feel "light" and makes them have the desire to move their bodies.

Many people fail in their attempts in doing exercise simply because they forget that in order to spend energy they have to have energy available in the first place.

The other most common cause of failure in a new exercise routine is the situation of LACK OF A GRADIENT. A "gradient" is a level, grade or power for something. For example, stairs are "gradients" in a staircase. The different temperatures of a thermometer are "gradients" of temperature. Gradients are important in life. First you crawl, then you walk and then you finally run. These are different gradients of actions of different intensities and they are necessary.

When overweight or obese people decide to start exercising, they are making the right decision. But they are going to be even more right and more successful with their knowledge and application of these factors. The first goal is to obtain more energy from their metabolism through food and some natural supplements that help increase energy levels. The second goal is to choose an

APPROPRIATE GRADIENT for the level of exercise. If a person expects to be able to run a marathon after having spent the last 20 years of their life working in front of a computer at the office and while lacking energy, they most definitely are going to add another failure to their list of previous failures.

The key is to start exercising after you have obtained more energy from your metabolism and to start doing exercise slowly on an appropriate intensity gradient, like walking, swimming or another type of exercise that isn't incredibly straining to a body that has been more accustomed to a sedentary lifestyle. For example, if you initially do exercises that cause a lot of muscular pain, the gradient is too intense for your body. If someone decides to walk and walks so fast that they have trouble breathing they are walking too quickly for their current respiratory ability. Exercising on the right gradient doesn't cause severe muscular pain or trouble breathing. More people fail because they select an improper exercise gradient that is too intense for their "out of shape" body than for any other reason. The "desperation" or "rush" that we have when we start a new workout routine is always the root cause of the eventual failure.

The way in which exercise gives results is by increasing the gradient little by little. Say we start with 15 minutes a day, 4 days a week. The following week we go up to 20 minutes of exercise, and keep on increasing little by little, to give your body the opportunity to get used to the routine. In no time you will have improved your physical condition, but by using GRADIENTS.

Any exercise is good when it comes to increasing your metabolism. My favorite, without having to buy any kind of special equipment, is walking. I recommend that people initially only walk until they come to a slight sweat. It is at this point where the metabolism has been increased enough to create the heat that caused the sweat. The metabolism generates heat and the heat provokes sweat. The point where your body starts to sweat is the point where you have already succeeded in increasing your metabolism with exercise.

However, I should mention that there is an exercise that in my experience works better than all others in boosting your metabolism. It is an exercise in which you bounce on a small trampoline to the rhythm of music.

I have never seen an exercise help people lose weight more quickly than bouncing on a small trampoline. I spent many years researching different kinds of exercise that could help overweight or obese people, taking into consideration that these people don't have large amounts of energy or strength. I saw that some exercises are definitely not appropriate for overweight people because they are exercises like jogging, which can cause damage on the knees or weight lifting, which can hurt the back. Other exercises have the main disadvantage of being boring, like walking on a treadmill or lifting weights. Some require a lot of space, or specialized equipment like exercise bikes or swimming pools.

Bouncing on a small trampoline is a low impact exercise that any overweight or obese person can do. It doesn't require much strength because the trampoline absorbs the resistance of the bounce. According to the studies I've seen, trampolines have the main benefit of exercising the ENTIRE body due to the bouncing motion and of going against and then in favor of gravity while also stimulating and exercising all of the cells of the body without exception.

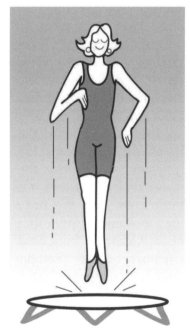

This type of exercise works out ALL of the cells in your body. The body's cells, with their coordinated actions, are the ones that generate the metabolism or the energy of the body. When all of them are exercised, they are stimulated to increase the metabolism.

My experience is that doing this exercise for just 15 minutes made my body keep on sweating for more than an hour (1) after having stopped, which indicated to me that I had successfully and noticeably increased my metabolism. After three weeks of doing the bouncing exercise for just 15 minutes, 3 days a week, I had to go to a tailor to have all of my clothes adjusted and that made it obvious that this exercise really reduces a good amount of the body's fat.

There is a scientific reason as to why exercising on the trampoline seems to be much more effective than other exercises in helping people increase their metabolism and lose weight. It has to do with the design of the body. The human body eliminates toxins and fats through what is called the lymphatic system. The lymphatic system is composed of tiny ducts. These ducts are so small that blood doesn't fit in them. An off-white liquid flows through the lymphatic system that is called lymph. The body disposes and gets rid of the toxins of the cells and the fats in this liquid, the lymph. We could say that the lymphatic system is the body's drainage system. It is the system that the body uses to eliminate what isn't needed anymore from what 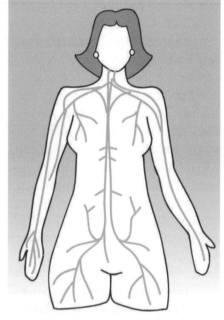 is left over from the reactions inside the cells. The lymphatic system doesn't have a pump that pushes this liquid, the lymph, like in the case of the blood's circulatory system where our heart serves as a pressure pump. The lymph moves with gravity and with the help of the body's movements. The bouncing movement on the small trampoline that moves with and against gravity moves the lymph fluid and extracts the body's toxins from the cells and also the fat. This is why this type of exercise in particular helps a lot in increasing your metabolism and decreasing the fat in your body.

What I liked the most about bouncing on the trampoline was that it was enjoyable; I didn't find myself bored like I did with other types of exercise. Bouncing to the music without feeling an impact on my knees and bouncing to the rhythm, the 15 minutes of exercise went much faster than any other exercise that I had done before.

There are various books written in reference to this bouncing exercise, as well as studies done by NASA that show its effectiveness is superior to other exercises like jogging or running on a treadmill. NASA uses trampolines to exercise the astronauts when they return from space missions because it helps them regain their balance and recuperate their muscles after a prolonged period of being in space without gravity.

Physical exercise, of any kind, has an added benefit that will help you. Physical exercise significantly lowers the effects of daily stress. When we are stressed, our body produces a lot of *cortisol* and this hormone doesn't only make us fat in the abdomen and hips, it also doesn't allow us to sleep well. *Cortisol* is a hormone that causes insomnia and sleeping problems. The combination of an abundance of stress, a large amount of *cortisol* and lack of good sleep is one of the main obstacles in losing weight. People that don't sleep well also don't lose weight because they have levels of *cortisol* that are too high. When we exercise, the body gets rid of a good amount of the *cortisol* that is accumulated from the stress experienced during the day through the liver and that's why after doing exercise we always sleep much better and wake up feeling rested.

So, if you want to improve your metabolism you have to exercise. Nevertheless, make sure that you first increase your energy production level by improving your diet before going and spending energy that you don't have. After you have acquired more energy to invest in your exercises make sure you start on an appropriate exercise gradient so that you are successful in your attempt and feel good about yourself.

TIME TO RECOVER YOUR METABOLISM

YOUR MIND CONTROLS EVERYTHING

Successes or failures always come from some action and all actions are born from a decision. In any project we take on, the most important thing is to have the DECISION.

Many people who have experienced a slow metabolism have tried numerous times to lose weight only to find they fail very shortly after starting. What keeps a person enthusiastic about achieving their goal are RESULTS. If a person tries to lose weight and doesn't succeed, they will add yet another failed experience. Many consecutive failure experiences lead a person to a state of emotional apathy (the thought that "no effort is worth it"). From an emotional state of apathy, we then give rise to the justifications phrases of those people that are tired of failing. Phrases like "I am happy being fat" or "This is the way I am, and this is the way I'll always be".

The first factor to consider is the factor of the problem itself, the "slow metabolism". Logic says that someone who doesn't know mathematics will never be able to solve an algebraic equation. In the same sense, someone who knows nothing or very little about the causes and possible solutions to a slow metabolism will fail in any attempt they make. You can't solve a problem that you don't understand! So, the first logical step in resolving any problem is by understanding it. If you don't understand the factors that create a "slow metabolism" you also won't be able to solve it because you would be "working blindly" against the problem. The logical solution is to increase your KNOWLEDGE of the problem to be able to solve it.

So, if you are one of those people who have tried "thousands of diets", miracle pills, gym memberships, starving yourself, counting calories, acupuncture, mesotherapy [22] or some other method, you have to realize that you never had the KNOWLEDGE on how to do it and that is why you failed. It's not that you have "lack of willpower" or that you lack discipline. Anyone that makes a huge effort and sacrifices to lose weight and doesn't see results will give up after trying for so long. If you didn't give up, you wouldn't be human. All efforts deserve a reward. If you make the effort and never receive the reward you obviously can't go on.

The difference between success and failure is always the KNOWLEDGE about the obstacles and the possible solutions. We have been discussing the different factors that cause a slow metabolism and now you know them. At this point you should have found which ones apply directly to you and you should have some sort of plan to manage them. And now you also have the KNOWLEDGE and therefore you can succeed.

It is the mind that controls the body. The body seldom controls the mind. Being able to use your mind to make correct decisions is your most valuable ability.

There is a mental exercise that will help you make the right decisions and focus on your new goal of increasing your metabolism, losing weight, and later maintaining a weight that suits you for the rest of your life.

The exercise can be done on a piece of paper. Start out by writing a list of ALL the attempts you remember having made to lose weight or get in shape throughout your whole life. This list, in some cases, can be very long and would look something like this:

---

[22] Mesotherapy – A medical therapy that uses multiple injections of pharmaceutical and homeopathic medications, plant extracts, vitamins and other ingredients to break the body's fat.

ATTEMPTS TO LOSE WEIGHT OR GET IN SHAPE

Atkins Diet	Acupuncture
Calorie Diet	Naturalist doctor
Vegetarian Diet	Orlistat (Alli)
Nutritionist	Treadmill
Hydroxycut	Hypnosis treatment
Soup Diet	Gym membership
Herbalife	Grapefruit Diet
Jenny Craig	Live food Diet
LA Weight Loss	Homeopathic drops
Bariatric doctor	Adipex
Weight Watchers	Walking in the park
Overeaters Anonymous	Slim Fast shakes

Making a list while trying to remember EVERYTHING that you have ever tried to lose weight or get in shape will help you analyze the different efforts you have made. Some of the things that you have done will surely seem like truly unfounded hopes on your part.

Now comes the most important and powerful part of the mental exercise. Locate in your mind what your MAIN PURPOSE was behind all of your efforts and write it on the paper. In other words, a phrase of yours that expresses what you wanted to achieve. That PURPOSE that moved you to spend God knows how much money and effort on all of those failed attempts.

The MAIN PURPOSE is very personal and only yours. We are all different and we all have different MAIN PURPOSES. For example, the MAIN PURPOSE for one person could be "to lose weight to look better", while another "to feel healthy" or someone else "to be able to wear the clothes I have hanging in my closet" and, for others, things like "to look as beautiful as when I first got married". Whatever your MAIN PURPOSE was, the important thing is that you find it and write it on a piece of paper. The only purpose that is important is your purpose; your MAIN PURPOSE.

Once you have found what your true MAIN PURPOSE was, have it written down, and are sure that it is really what motivated you, now comes the IMPORTANT question that you must ask yourself:

Do I still want to achieve my main purpose?

If your answer to this question is YES, we have restored your MAIN PURPOSE and you can now achieve it this time. Your mind controls everything. In finding your main purpose and deciding that it is still something that you really want to attain, an important phenomenon has happened: your main purpose has been restored in your mind.

If the answer to the question is NO, you will have to dedicate a bit of time to finding out what your own personal MAIN PURPOSE is with regards to this topic of the metabolism and losing weight. For example, a purpose like "lose weight to please my husband" is not your own purpose; it's your husband's purpose. If you try to lose weight based on someone else's purpose you will for sure fail. If you don't find your own MAIN PURPOSE that is really your own purpose, don't even try! Without a very clear and strong purpose in your mind you will surely fail again.

In order to be successful in any aspect of life, we must have a clear goal for our action and that is what a "purpose" is. This is why a young man who studies for a certain profession to "please his mother" generally graduates with good grades and ends up working at a job that has nothing to do with what he studied. The subject that he studied wasn't his desire (purpose), but his mother's. This fact is so basic that it applies to everything that we do in life including losing weight.

There isn't anything that is more powerful than your mind. If you think you can, you can. If you decide that you are going to "try", you have already failed. The power of your intention and clearly finding your purpose makes the difference.

Take into consideration that on the path toward your goal you will run into moments of difficulty. Only your perseverance will make you prevail. "Where there's a will, there's a way" is very true, but you have to really want to achieve your goal. It has to be a firm and final decision that you make that you are going to achieve what you set out to do.

LOSE WEIGHT OR SLIM DOWN?

Throughout the years nothing has been as arduous as convincing all of the people who seek out help at NaturalSlim that what they really want to do is "slim down". The public mind is dominated by the wrong idea of "losing weight".

I have spent many long hours convincing people that the important thing is not to "lose weight"; the important thing is to slim down, which means, "reducing your body fat". There is a difference!

The human body is composed of many things: flesh, bones, nerves, muscles, water, fat, minerals, etc. The general public that is seeking help has this obsession with "losing weight". People torment themselves with their goals of "losing weight". However, the problem with us, as a population, isn't that we weigh a lot. The problem with us is that we are fat. Our bodies are way too full of fat.

The difference here is that what we really want to do is reduce our body FAT. We don't want to reduce the water, bones or muscles of the body, just the FAT. In other words, we want to "slim down".

I myself use "lose weight" and "slim down" interchangeably throughout this book. I have gotten used to "losing weight" because it is what everyone else has in his or her mind. However, what we really need to do is SLIM DOWN.

Many of the people following this wrong goal of "losing weight" have done permanent damage to their bodies. For example, not too long ago I met a 17-year-old young woman that had a deformed body with her skin hanging and falling off of her abdomen, arms and even her face. This young woman, who was only 17 years old, looked like she was at least 25. She had aged prematurely. The young woman in question had experienced severe depression due to her obesity and her decision had been to "lose weight". In fact, she lost 80 pounds, but did it with an inhumane diet in which she only ate cabbage soup three times a day for ten months. She lost 80 pounds but, in the process, caused so much starvation to her body, that a significant amount of her muscles was destroyed. Since muscles are what hold the skin in place, destroying her muscles caused all of her skin to sag and it deformed her young body. The damage is permanent.

What you want to do is "slim down". We don't want to destroy the muscles in our body because our muscles are what hold our skin in place like tension cables. If we starve our bodies, our muscles will be destroyed, and our skin will start to sag. If the skin sags, then only plastic surgery can help us, and we will never achieve what was possible if we had done things right in the first place.

If you decide to slim down, you must forget about your weight. Weight will be lost but what is IMPORTANT is that you lower your FAT. When the fat is reduced you will notice the change in your clothing size and if you are a man you will notice it in your waistline. This is what is important, lowering your clothing size! If your clothing size or your waistline is becoming smaller, that tells you that you are doing it right; you are reducing your body's FAT.

The majority of people have a serious misunderstanding about fat. Fat is not a heavy substance. In fact, fat is the lightest thing in your body! What really weigh a lot are water, muscles and bones.

If you look closely you will be able to notice, when at the beach or in the swimming pool, that people who have more fat in their bodies float much easier, while skinny people can't float much at all. Fat is so light that it floats. The problem is that fat is a VOLUMINOUS substance. In other words, it is a substance that occupies a lot of space. But, fat has never been a heavy substance.

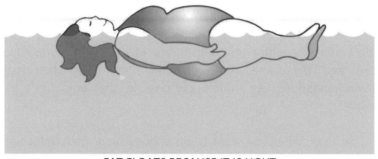

FAT FLOATS BECAUSE IT IS LIGHT

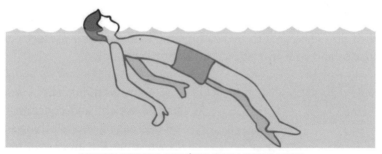

SKINNY PEOPLE DON'T FLOAT VERY EASILY

For example, when people work out, their muscular mass increases and thus so does their weight. The people working out will have increased their muscle mass while reducing body fat; therefore, they will weigh more because of the added muscles and at the same time be slenderer.

A while ago I was talking with a NaturalSlim client that had went from a size 22 to a size 8 using our services. She was very happy. She was telling me about her current exercise routine along with what techniques she was using to increase her metabolism that she had learned from us. She told me that she had once been on another "weight loss" plan where they didn't allow exercise. She told me that they didn't allow exercise because "exercise increases your weight".

I was almost in a state of shock hearing this. How could someone possibly recommend to another person who wants to boost his or her metabolism and become slender that they not work out because it would make them gain weight? I realized that the misunderstanding between "losing weight" and "slimming down" didn't only exist with public consumers. Many health professionals have had the same confusion and that's why they make recommendations like "don't exercise so that you don't gain weight".

So then, what you want to do is boost your metabolism and SLIM DOWN. Forget about your damn weight! What good will it do for you to "lose weight" if your clothes still fitted you more and more tightly? What you really want to watch is your clothing size or your waistline. You want your fat to go away and not have your skin hang off of you like rags. To avoid this, it is vital that you protect your muscles and your hydration. You want to slim down.

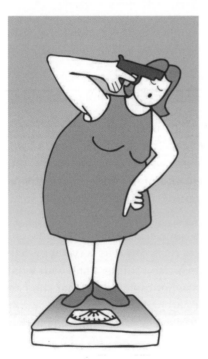

Stop worrying about your body's weight and concentrate on decreasing your clothing size or waistline. Put away your scale so that you don't get anxious by weighing yourself all the time. If you cause a stressful situation by trying to "lose weight" you won't be able to slim down because you will have caused a large production of the stress hormone, *cortisol. Cortisol* is a hormone that makes you gain weight and doesn't allow you to slim down. Don't try to slim down by stressing yourself out or pushing yourself to extremes to "lose weight" because you will already have sabotaged your efforts.

If someone notices that you are slimming down and asks you the usual — "how much weight have you lost?" — tell him or her that your problem never was being "heavy". Your problem was being a little bit "fat" and therefore you are only interested in reducing the fat in your body; that's why you don't make it a custom to weigh yourself. If you want, tell them what clothing size you've went down to or how many inches you've lost off your waistline. In the process you will teach the person a lesson about "slimming down" as opposed to "losing weight".

Also take note that you shouldn't have unrealistic expectations. If you suffer from various health conditions you will always have a more difficult time slimming down than if you were in perfect health. Say you have high blood pressure, asthma, diabetes, hypothyroidism or another condition; that reflects that your body is not in an optimum state. A healthy body slims down easily. An unhealthy body slims down slowly.

As for expectations, you should also be aware that a younger body has more potential to recover the metabolism and slim down. The contrary is also true. For example, at my age, 57, I have to put forth much more effort. I have to be much more disciplined in my lifestyle than a young man who is only 25 years old would have to be.

Women always slim down slower than men. Don't think about getting into a competition to slim down with your husband. The reason is that men have much more muscle (about 40% more) than women. Since muscle is what burns fat, men always slim down faster than women.

The important thing to remember is what we want: to increase our metabolism and "slim down".

YOUR BODY IS ALIVE

It seems silly to have to say it, but "your body is alive". The point here is that live organisms have certain characteristics and abilities that are very different than things that are dead. The human body is an organism that is alive. What you need to know is that since your body is alive, it has the ability to learn and adapt.

It is calculated that human bodies have lived on this planet for the last 75 million years. That is a long time. Throughout all this time the conditions in the environment, the food and the lives of human beings have suffered many changes. Human bodies have been able to survive all of these eras simply because they are organisms that learn and adapt.

We need to be aware of our body's abilities to learn to adapt when we decide to increase our metabolism and slim down. If you don't take it into account, you could fail in your attempt. Your body adapts to everything. It adapts to your diet, to being starved, to not drinking water, to sleeping too little or to whatever else we make it go through.

In fact, the reason that the diets of counting calories don't work is due to the same fact; bodies learn and adapt. When a person goes on a diet of counting calories in reality what they are really trying to do is to lower the sources of energy for their body. Diets of counting calories are diets, in many cases, of "starving out" by simply eating less than what you'd like to eat. They don't work.

The reason that diets of counting calories don't work is due to the fact that the body is alive, and it feels the drastic reduction of food that these diets bring about. In the beginning, the person starts losing weight when they do this type of diet. Their main weight loss in the first two weeks will be loss of water. Later, the person continues the diet and starts losing weight but notices that each week that goes by their weight loss is less. In other words, something happened that made their metabolism slower.

Well, what has been discovered about this is that the body "learns" and "adapts" to the decreased availability of food, decreasing the metabolism. The body interprets the reduction of food as a condition of "shortage". Its' solution to the "shortage" is to slow down the metabolism, which in turn, slows down the function of the thyroid gland.

This decrease of your metabolism has been proven, by measuring the production of the T3 hormone that the thyroid gland produces while a person is dieting. The T3 hormone is an "active" hormone that determines the speed or rate of your metabolism. The longer that a person is on a diet, the larger the decrease of their available T3 hormone will be. It's your body's adaptation mechanism. Eating less food equals having a slower metabolism. It is your body's attempt to "economize" in times of "shortage".

In other words, reduced calorie diets give your body the wrong message. They give the message that it has to decrease your metabolism because if it doesn't it will go hungry. Since the body is designed to survive, its response to a decrease in the food supply is to reduce the function of the thyroid gland and therefore also the metabolism, in order to be able to survive with less food. It is an adaptation reaction of your body.

Some people ask themselves why it is so difficult for them to lose weight even when they are "going hungry". That is the reason. When you force your body to "go hungry" you are making it adapt to the shortage of food and the body must reduce the function of the thyroid and metabolism to protect itself.

The problem here is that the body "learns" from you. This learning turns into a type of "cellular memory" under which the body's cells "remember" the moments of shortage and adapt to having a slower metabolism. If you insist on convincing your body that there is a food shortage, your body will keep on decreasing your metabolism to "economize". The cells will remember these moments of shortage. This is the beginning of the famous "slow metabolism". If you teach your body that in order to survive it has to consume less food, it will not have any other choice but to reduce the metabolism to be able to survive the hunger and shortage that you have caused it. It is suicide for the metabolism.

What would you do if one day you heard on the news that there was a shortage of food in every supermarket in the country? Wouldn't you take some sort of action to save the food that you have in your house or try to buy more food while the crisis lasts? Well, if there is a shortage, your body does exactly the same thing you would do: economize and store! The way that your body economizes is by reducing the metabolism through the thyroid gland. The way that your body stores energy is by accumulating fat.

When someone has done one of those diets of counting calories that make them starve or one of those drastic diets of only eating soup for several days, the body finds itself obligated to decrease the metabolism. The moment when you abandon the diet, your body will be eagerly ready, waiting to store the food that you give it; and it is going to save it as fat. This is because the body will be adapting to store energy (fat) in order to prepare for the next time the "shortage" happens. This is the reason for the so-called "bounce" or "yo-yo effect" of the traditional diets of "eating less" or "counting calories".

When you do a diet of eating fewer calories you are creating a "slow metabolism" and your body keeps on adapting to the situation. When you finally give up the diet and try to eat normal portions of food, your body, which already has a slow metabolism, will begin to accumulate and save fat. It is an attempt that your body makes to get ready to survive the next diet of "going hungry" that you impose on it.

There are some differences that must be established. Your body is alive. You are a being that inhabits your body. You are not your body. You have thoughts and feelings and you make decisions. Your body doesn't actually think, nor does it make decisions or have emotions. You are you and your body is your body. You and your body are not the same thing.

We'd like to think that it is you that controls your body (we hope) and not your body that controls you. But, you can't forget that the body is a living organism and that live organisms learn and adapt to their environment and to the conditions that they confront. Don't make the mistake of giving your body the message that there is a food shortage. If you do that, you will have a "slow metabolism", and it will make slimming down difficult or impossible to do.

In my experience, people that have made the most random, drastic dieting attempts to lose weight are the people with the "slowest metabolisms". In other words, the people that have been "on a diet their entire life" and go from one popular diet to the next, are the people that have done the most damage to their metabolism. They have successfully convinced their body that there is a constant food shortage. Your body's solution, since living organisms learn and adapt, has been to decrease the metabolism to be able to survive the shortages.

So then, to be able to increase your metabolism all you have to do is reverse the body's process of learning and adapting. In my experience, it is much easier to convince the body to slow down the metabolism than it is to speed it up. The reasons can be found within the section about the thyroid gland (see the topic PROBLEMS WITH THE THYROID GLAND SYSTEM).

What is important is that you understand that there is a very close connection between what you do with your body and the reactions your body has. If you aren't aware of the fact that your body is alive, you won't know what actions of yours give it the right message: increase the metabolism, and what actions of yours force it to reduce the metabolism. Yes, your body is alive.

FOODS: SOURCES OF ENERGY FOR THE METABOLISM

The metabolism is the sum of all of the movements, actions and changes that your body does, to convert food and nutrients into energy in order to survive. The metabolism is an energy conversion system. Food and nutrients (vitamins, minerals and water) are sources of energy like the gas that you put in your car. The metabolism turns these energy sources into energy to breathe, move, protect, grow and survive.

Foods are sources of energy. However, in the same way that there are different levels of octane (potencies) of gasoline, there are also different types of foods that have different levels of potential energy for your body.

Natural carbohydrates (vegetables and salad) that aren't starches provide energy for a short amount of time (3-4 hours) and are very clean foods, very complete in nutrients and very good for you. Notice that when you eat only a salad for lunch you feel hungry again much earlier in the afternoon than if you had eaten a meal with meat (protein) for lunch.

Starches (potato, sweet potato, cassava, yams, parsnip and other root vegetables) provide energy for a short period of time and have many good nutrients. Starches are also by definition "simple sugars" (as defined in the dictionary), which quickly turn into glucose. This means you can't abuse them because if you consume them in large portions you will gain weight.

Refined carbohydrates (sugar, bread, flour, pasta, rice, crackers, etc.) provide a very short-term amount of energy (2-3 hours). Refined carbohydrates are foods that have already been cooked, polished, smashed, filtered or processed in some other way industrially. The molecules of these foods are already very small and that means that they are absorbed very quickly with very little work of your digestive system. That's why your body can turn them into glucose at a rate that is "faster than fast". The excess glucose, as you already know, along with the excess insulin that it creates, is the cause of weight and obesity problems.

Refined carbohydrates bring along with them another critical problem: they are deprived of nutrients (vitamins and minerals). It's what nutritionists call "empty calories". The industrial processes that refined carbohydrates are put through strip them of the majority of their vitamins and minerals, which make them an "non-food". In other words, they are foods that don't provide nourishment. In order for the body to be able to turn food into energy to increase the metabolism, it is forced to use the vitamins and minerals that the foods contain. If the food barely has any vitamins and minerals, the food only serves to create more glucose and with the help of insulin will then create: more fat.

People that have emigrated from countries in the Caribbean, Central or South America, such as the Dominican Republic, Venezuela or Mexico, are surprised at how quickly they gain weight in the United States. This phenomenon is easy to understand when we compare the type of carbohydrates that they consumed in their countries as opposed to the refined carbohydrates that predominate here. The refined carbohydrates that we consume here are deprived of vitamins and minerals; they really make you gain weight. As if this wasn't enough, our refined carbohydrates contain dyes and preservatives that decrease the metabolism. The carbohydrates that they ate in their native countries were much less industrialized and their bodies weren't forced to turn them into fat.

Proteins (meat, seafood, cheese, eggs) are foods that we could call "high octane", high potency foods. Proteins take a lot more time to digest and their energy production in the body lasts much longer (4-6 hours). That is why you will find it difficult to eat an early dinner after eating a lunch that was high in proteins, because you will still feel full.

I should mention that just as there are different qualities of gasoline, there are also different qualities of proteins, like meats. Meats that help you slim down the most are white meats like chicken, turkey, fish and seafood. Red meats (beef and pork) have a disadvantage in that they contain a compound called *arachidonic acid* (AA) that tends to cause inflammation in the body. This doesn't mean that you have to completely eliminate all red meat from your diet. It's just that if you want to boost your metabolism as much as possible, you should lower your portions of red meat and prefer white meat over red. If you do this, slimming down will happen much faster. This isn't to say that you can't reward yourself with a pork chop or some ribs every once in a while, if you enjoy them. It is a question of choosing those meats that increase the metabolism the most. All the substances that produce or promote inflammations in the body, like the *arachidonic acid* (AA) that red meat has, will tend to decrease the speed of the metabolism.

Fats are foods that provide a lot of energy. They are foods that provide a sense of fullness and satisfaction. Their effect of energy production is similar to that of proteins (4-6 hours). When you eat fat or oils with your food, you feel full faster because the fats and oils provoke a reaction in your body that produces the CCK hormone. The CCK hormone is really called *"cholecystokinin"* or *"pancreozymin"*. It is a hormone that the body produces in response to the fats and oils, it is the hormone that sends the message to the brain that "I'm full, I'm not hungry anymore". In studies that have been done of injecting the CCK hormone into different animals, it always caused hunger to disappear.

This is the same reason why diets that are low in fat have uncomfortable feelings of hunger, due to a lack of the CCK hormone production that they cause. For example, as you will learn further on in the book, organic coconut oil is saturated fats that will dramatically reduce hunger and will make you slim down. This is because this oil provokes a strong reaction of the CCK hormone and your body will simply stop feeling hungry.

The ideal diet to increase your metabolism should contain fats and oils. Fats can be saturated like the fat in pork meat, but pork is a meat that you shouldn't abuse. The best fats to slim down are the fats and oils found in fish and seafood. Olive oil is also an excellent option for you.

When you consume saturated fats like those contained in pork meat, you should avoid combining them with a high consumption of refined carbohydrates at all costs. If you combine saturated fats with refined carbohydrates, you will have created a real nutritional disaster for your body. You have to remember that refined carbohydrates provoke a high production of insulin in your body. The insulin hormone will help your body convert both the fats and the carbohydrates that you ate into additional stored fat for your body. If you combine saturated fats with natural carbohydrates like salad or vegetables, like say pork chops with salad, you will still be able to lose weight because there wouldn't be enough insulin produced to make you fat.

Fiber is part of carbohydrates and is highly recommended. That's why, if you are going to eat bread, it would be better if you get a whole wheat bread that is high in fiber. In general, the whiter the bread is, the less fiber it will have. Breads that are high in fiber are never white or light colored. In Europe, you'll find that people eat a type of bread that is very hard to chew. This is because in Europe people like bread that is high in fiber and therefore the breads are very hard in texture and in consistency. Obesity in Europe isn't even half of the problem that we have on our side of the world where the bread is white, sweet and soft.

Each type of food contributes to the metabolism in a different way. Nothing is or should be forbidden; nothing. However, here the logical goal is to consume more of those foods that help speed up the metabolism and less of those that slow it down.

THE POTENCY OF YOUR VITAMINS IS IMPORTANT

THIS IS VITAL INFORMATION

In order to boost your metabolism, there are thousands of internal body processes and chemical reactions that must happen so that the body can carry out an extraction of energy from the foods and nutrients that you eat. If these internal chemical processes and changes in your body don't perform efficiently, your body will produce very little energy and will continue having a "slow metabolism".

To extract the energy that foods contain and turn it into useable energy for the metabolism, the human body uses more than 500 different enzymes. The enzymes themselves, in turn, depend on specific vitamins and minerals to be able to do their job.

Modern medical authorities have tried to play down the importance of supplementing your diet with vitamins and minerals. They claim that "there isn't sufficient evidence" to prove that there are vitamin or mineral deficiencies amongst our population. Oddly enough, there was a recent study that showed that less than 20% of doctors recommend that their patients take a daily vitamin or mineral supplement. However, the same study revealed that 56% (the majority) of doctors personally take some sort of daily supplement of vitamins. It's a professional attitude of "it's not necessary" along with the personal attitude of "let me take them just in case".

I can tell you that from the experience of working with thousands of people, if you don't take high potency vitamin and mineral supplements, you will not successfully increase your metabolism nor slim down at a decent speed. It's the truth, without potent vitamins, you won't make it. And if the vitamins that you take are the commercial types that are low potency, like the vitamins put out by *Centrum*, you won't succeed, either.

You see, vitamins vary by the potency of their dose. Commercial vitamins like *Centrum* and various others only contain 1 or 2 milligrams of the B complex vitamins (B-1, B-2, B-3, B-5, and B-6). Good potency vitamins contain 25 to 50 milligrams of each one of the B vitamins. In other words, they are 25 to 50 times more potent than the commercial ones.

One area where you shouldn't try to save or "cut corners" is in your selection of a good potency multivitamin formula. If you buy cheap vitamins that are low potency, you can apply the phrase "being cheap is expensive" because you will not overcome your "slow metabolism". You will have lost your time again and you will have to add another failure to your long list. Without strong vitamins and minerals you will not succeed.

When you go to buy vitamins pay attention to the dosage size per each vitamin or mineral that the formula contains. High potency vitamins never have less than 25 milligrams of each one of the B complex vitamins. The B complex vitamins are the ones that control the production of energy in your body. Without them, your body will not be able to produce enough energy to be able to boost your metabolism.

When you take high potency multivitamins and minerals every day, you feel a difference. With commercial vitamins, you don't feel a difference.

There are several vitamins and minerals that are closely related to the processes of your metabolism. Many years of having consumed a poor diet high in refined carbohydrates produces an accumulation of deficiencies that affects the production of energy down to the cellular level. Generally, the more overweight or obese a person is, the more vitamin and mineral deficiencies they will have.

On the other hand, there are various medications for diabetes, high blood pressure, heart disease and various other conditions that cause a vitamin deficiency in your body. To mention a few of them, aspirin causes vitamin C and B-12 deficiencies. Vitamin B-12 is essential for hemoglobin[23], which are the cells that transport oxygen to your body cells. The condition where one has low hemoglobin is called anemia. The same thing happens with medications that are used to control high cholesterol which actually deplete certain vitamins and minerals in the body.

Some vitamin and mineral deficiencies directly impact the functioning of the thyroid gland that controls your body's metabolism. For example, the thyroid produces the T4 hormone but this hormone isn't an active hormone until an enzyme called *deiodinase* converts the T4 into the T3 hormone. The enzyme *deiodinase* completely depends on the mineral called selenium[24]. This is why it has been found that all the people that are hypothyroid are also deficient in this mineral, selenium.

The thyroid gland can't manufacture the T4 hormone if it doesn't have enough of the minerals zinc or copper. The body needs very small amounts of these minerals but missing even these small amounts will make it impossible for the thyroid gland to produce the needed T4 hormone if it lacks zinc, copper, or selenium.

---

[23] Hemoglobin: blood cells that transport oxygen to the rest of the cells in the body. When the hemoglobin is too low one develops a condition called "anemia".

[24] Selenium – is a mineral of which trace (very small) amounts are necessary for cellular function in most, if not all, animals, forming the active center of certain enzymes.

For the body trying to produce thyroid hormones without having zinc, copper or selenium is like trying to construct a building without having any cement.

On the other hand, a diabetic's insulin is impossible to make when there is a deficiency of the mineral magnesium. Many diabetics are diabetic due to their bodies producing an insulin hormone that seems to be defective and it creates a condition called "insulin resistance". As soon as they start taking a high potency multivitamin and minerals formula, diabetics notice that their blood glucose levels start to go down and become easier to control. With their body getting the vitamins and minerals that it needs, it stops producing the defective insulin hormone and this contributes to the normalizing of their blood sugar (glucose).

Within the subject of the metabolism there are no miracles. Your body needs what it needs to be able to boost the metabolism. If you give your body what it needs to function, you will see the results. Taking a high potency multivitamin and mineral formula every day is vital for success.

HOW IS BODY FAT MADE?

To be able to slim down you must understand how fat is created in your body. The idea is that a person speeds up the rate of their metabolism to "burn" their excess body fat while avoiding the accumulation of new fat. That's why you HAVE to know how new fat is created in your body; so that you can avoid it.

Fat is necessary. It is a substance that protects our organs, protects us from the cold and stores within itself lots of potential energy. If a time came when there was a serious food shortage, the first to die of starvation would be the "skinny" people, and the last would be obese people. When the body doesn't have any other choice, it uses its fat as a source of energy to survive. Bears hibernate for many months, and during this time their bodies are using their stored fat. That's why when bears start their hibernation they are fat and when they wake up they are very thin. Fat is a substance that stores energy for future use.

The process of the creation of body fat is the following:

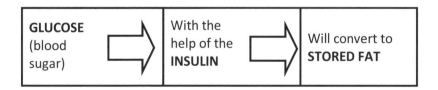

GLUCOSE (blood sugar)	With the help of the INSULIN	Will convert to STORED FAT

The reason that diets that are high in refined carbohydrates cause weight and obesity problems is because no other group of foods produces more glucose, more quickly, than refined carbohydrates. A large amount of glucose forces the body to produce a large quantity of the insulin hormone. If your body cells use the glucose that they need and end up having more than enough of it left over, the body will create fat to "store" the surplus of glucose.

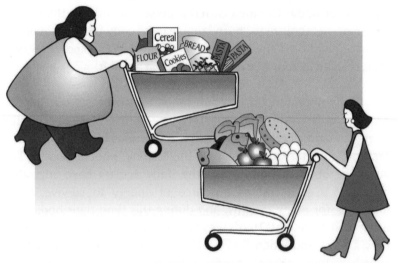

AN EXCESS OF REFINED CARBOHYDRATES LEADS TO WEIGHT AND OBESITY PROBLEMS

Proteins and fats also produce glucose, but they make it in very small amounts that don't stimulate a very high production of insulin. It is the insulin that allows us to gain weight. Insulin could be compared to a shopping cart in that it brings glucose along with it to the cells to feed them. If the shopping carts (insulin) stays packed full of glucose, then the insulin will turn this excess glucose into fat for storage. So, there it is, the cause of weight problems and obesity: an excess of glucose and insulin in your blood. This also accounts for the high incidence of diabetes and conditions like hypoglycemia (low blood sugar).

FATS ARE NOT TO BLAME!

The general population is becoming every day more and more overweight. However, studies done by the government and the food industry reveal that we have decreased our consumption of fats for the last 40 consecutive years. For example, a United States federal government study called NHANES (National Health and Nutrition Examination Study) showed that the annual average consumption of fat is 19% less than it was 40 years ago.

The era of products that are fat-free, low fat and dubbed with the prefix "lite" have been dominating the food market for nearly 3 decades. How is it possible that the statistics reveal we are eating less fat if we are fatter than we have ever been?

For many years we have been sold on the idea that it is fat that causes more fat. As consumers we have believed this concept to the point that today we consume less fat than ever before. The constant publicity has made us conscious of the reality that they want to instill in us: "fat is what makes you fat". However, this is only a half-truth.

A "half-truth" is something that is partly true but that is also not 100% true. It's like if our wife or husband were to say to us, "I love you", when in reality what they mean is "I love you if you do whatever I say and never what I tell you not to". Taking that "I love you" as if it were an absolute truth would be a serious mistake.

The information that fats make us gain weight is a "half-truth". It has enough truth since it has been accepted as truth for many years. But, today, the percentages of weight problems and obesity of the population show that this wasn't absolutely true. It was only partly true.

It's true that fat can make us fat. But for this to be possible, the insulin hormone must be present. Without insulin present, fat can't make us fatter.

For example, the original Eskimos were nomadic tribes. The food that Eskimos could eat was limited to what they could find in the North Pole region. In the North Pole, there isn't land to sow or grow any kinds of plants. In the North Pole there is only snow and ice. Eskimos always survived by hunting and fishing animals. A nomadic Eskimo always made his breakfast, lunch and dinner with whatever he could catch by hunting or fishing. They fed themselves on fish, seals, polar bears and caribou (a type of polar deer). As a result, the only things that the Eskimos ate were meat and animal fat. There weren't carbohydrates in the North Pole, only meat and the fat that was in the fish and animals.

Taking into account the diet high in fat that the Eskimos had, we would expect to find very fat people amongst them. However, there were never nomadic Eskimos who were overweight or obese.

There was a research scientist named Henry Stephenson who traveled to the North Pole between 1875 and 1876 and lived with the Eskimos for 2 years. During this time, Stephenson ate the same things the Eskimos did, meat and fat. Stephenson was very surprised by the fact that in those 2 years, in which he was eating only meat and fat, he lost more than 40 pounds and he was much slenderer. At that time, Stephenson wrote a book about his discovery of how the diet of meat and fat had decreased his body fat.

The Masai tribe in Africa has survived healthfully for many generations by living off of only their livestock for food. The Masai eat the meat of their livestock as well as their milk and blood. The Masai were always known and respected by other tribes as thin, well-built warriors. Some years ago, some scientists did cholesterol tests on them and found that none of the members of the tribe had abnormally high cholesterol levels.

Due to the way that the body functions, the fat contained in foods can't turn into body fat unless there is enough insulin present. Insulin is only produced in large quantities when we consume refined carbohydrates. Without the help of insulin, the fats that we eat can't build up in our bodies. This is why even greasy pork meat can only make us fat if we have it with some type of carbohydrate that forces our body to produce insulin. The greasy pork meat alone can't make us fat.

The fat we consume has not been the cause of weight and obesity problems. The problem has been caused by the combination of fats and refined carbohydrates. For example, having pizza (bread with fat) for lunch or dinner would be a sure way to accumulate body fat.

You can eat fats without it meaning that they are going to make you fat. What is not smart is combining fat with refined carbohydrates.

Combining refined carbohydrates with fat is a sure way to WORSEN WHAT IS ALREADY BAD. If you want to slim down, you have to understand that fat is not what makes you fat. Without the help of insulin, which is created when we eat a good amount of carbohydrates, fat can't make us fat. Enjoy your pork chops with a nice salad. They won't make you fat. But be careful if you like to eat them with French-fried potatoes.

A Diet You Can Live With

The diet isn't the only factor that you have to know about to boost your metabolism and slim down. We have seen that there are many factors that lower the metabolism (dehydration, medications, the *candida albicans* yeast, stress and others).

However, the diet that we follow is an important factor and is also a deciding factor of whether we are going to succeed or fail in our attempt to slim down. Therefore, it makes sense to have a clear idea of which diet would be best to increase your metabolism. The ideal diet would be the one in which we don't feel we are on a diet. Furthermore, it would also be nice if the type of diet we choose could be turned into a permanent lifestyle that allows us to maintain a slender and healthy body once we have successfully slimmed down. In other words, a diet that doesn't lead to the famous "bounce-back" or "rebound", that happens to the majority of people that do diets, where they generally gain back the weight they lost and then some.

I have developed a diet system that doesn't forbid anything and can be easy to follow if you have a general idea of which foods allow you to slim down and which foods make you fat. One key point is that your body can only gain weight when it produces enough insulin, so the goal of a diet should be to decrease your insulin production. Insulin is the hormone that transports glucose (blood sugar) and also transports the fat that we eat to our body fat. In other words, it is insulin, or the excess of it, brought about by an excessive consumption of refined carbohydrates, that creates weight and obesity problems.

For the purpose of simplifying things, we can divide foods into groups according to how much insulin they stimulate the body to create when we eat them. The foods that cause a small insulin reaction in your body are the ones that MAKE YOU SLIM DOWN. On the contrary, the foods that stimulate a large production of insulin in your body are the foods that MAKE YOU FAT. The basic principle is that we want to utilize a type of diet that helps us slim down and thus, for our purposes there are only two types of foods:

FOOD TYPES	EXAMPLES	EFFECTS ON THE BODY	TYPE
Food that produces a **SMALL INSULIN REACTION** in the body	meats, chicken, turkey, fish, sea food, cheese, eggs, most vegetables, vegetable juices, salad, almonds, nuts	SLIMMING	S
Food that produces a **LARGE INSULIN REACTION** in the body	bread, pasta, flour, rice, potatoes, starches, corn, root vegetables, cereals, sugar, candy, chocolates, milk, fruit juices, sugary soft drinks	FATTENING	F

If we choose as part of our diet more foods of those that cause a small insulin reaction (TYPE S) and less of those that cause a large insulin reaction (TYPE F), we will begin to lose weight. Any diet that lowers the body's production of insulin will lower your body fat. In other words, slim down.

The system that I recommend is one in which you won't spend a lot of time measuring portions, weighing food or counting calories or carbohydrates – it is a VISUAL SYSTEM of FOOD PORTIONS. You choose the portions that you are going to eat of each type of food (S or F) and you picture them on your plate.

I call this system the "2x1 DIET" or "3x1 DIET". The "2x1" stands for having 2 Type S (slimming) foods for every 1 portion of Type F (fattening) food that you eat. In other words, 2 portions of those foods make you slim down (S) and only 1 portion of the type (F). Your plate would look something like this:

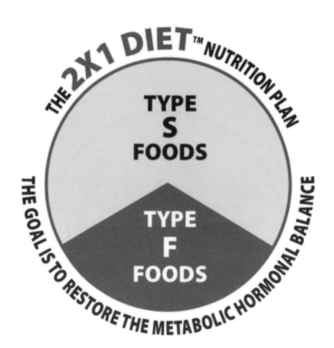

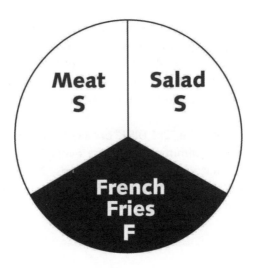

A way to understand it better is to look at the next photo of a plate of fried chicken (Type S), salad (Type S) and French fries (Type F). So, it's 2x1.

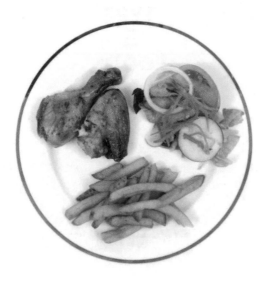

In the previous photo, perhaps you notice that there isn't very much food in the plate and you might think that you would still be hungry afterward. Just for the photo we put just a little bit of food on the plate so that you could clearly see the difference between the 3 types of foods. However, in the 2x1 diet you can eat enough of each one of these foods until you are fully satisfied. In fact, if you go hungry, your metabolism reduces, so we wouldn't recommend that you ever go hungry.

When you start the 2x1 Diet you'll notice that your hunger will go away. Your hunger goes away when you are on the 2x1 Diet because in eating less portions of Type F foods, your body produces less insulin. Insulin is the hormone that increases your hunger. In producing less insulin, you will have less feelings of hunger and you will feel full much faster and with less food.

For this diet system to work, you must consider EVERYTHING that you eat on this plate at the same time. In other words, if you decide to eat a good portion of the serving of bread before you have your main course, you don't then have the right to eat potatoes, which are Type F foods, because you already ate your portion of Type F foods in eating the bread. So, you choose what you want to eat, but make sure that the Type F foods are never more than a third of what you eat in whole. This is how you reduce the production of insulin in your body and start to slim down.

If, in place of potatoes or bread, you want to have a dessert, don't eat the bread or potatoes, so that you can leave your Type F portion for dessert. Then, you'll eat meat, salad and dessert, a 2x1 proportion between Type S (slimming) foods and Type F (fattening) foods.

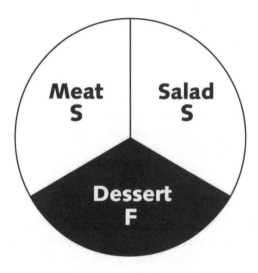

In this 2x1 Diet system you don't have to refuse anything. If you want, you can combine the Type F foods portion by eating only one slice of bread, a little bit of the potatoes and half of a dessert. The idea is that the sum of all of the Type F foods, which are really what make you fat from the high production of insulin that they cause, are never more than a third of what you consume in total. So, two portions of Type S (slimming) foods for one portion of a Type F food (fattening) are a "2x1".

The fat that is contained in the meat or protein will never make you fat if you make sure that your body's insulin production is low. You can achieve this by consuming controlled portions of the Type F foods. Without the help of insulin, the fat that you eat can't make you fat. It is the insulin that allows the fat that you consume to be used to produce more body fat. Without insulin, the fat that you eat simply can't make you fat. The trick is to control your body's production of insulin by managing your portions of Type F foods.

For example, if you eat a pork chop with salad, the fat from the meat can't be used by your body since, the salad caused a very small insulin reaction. But, if you make the mistake of eating a pork chop with a large portion of mashed potatoes, you are definitely going to gain fat. The mashed potatoes, being a starch that easily converts to glucose, will stimulate your body to produce a large amount of insulin and that is a sure way to become fatter. Insulin is the "shopping cart" that picks up the fat and glucose that then converts into new body fat. If you control your consumption of Type F foods you won't have problems with eating any type of fatty meat or other protein (cheese, eggs).

If you have a lot of fat to lose, if you are in a rush to slim down, or if you are a diabetic, then use the 3x1 Diet. In the 3x1, you make sure that the Type F foods are never more than a fourth of your total consumption. An example would be a meal that starts with a shrimp cocktail and is followed by a chicken breast with baked vegetables and a slice of bread.

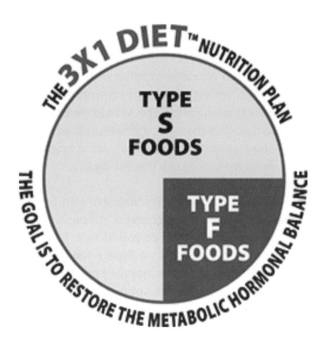

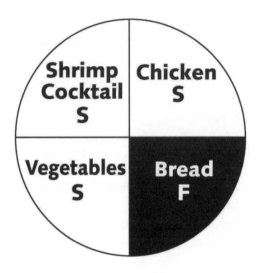

This above would be a 3x1. So, 3 portions of Type S foods are eaten for every portion of Type F foods.

The 3x1 diet produces less insulin in your body than the 2x1 for obvious reasons; it has a smaller portion of the Type F foods. For diabetics, the 3x1 is perfect because it controls glucose levels and helps them control their diabetes. The 3x1 also reduces the need for insulin for those diabetics that give themselves injections. Diabetics that measure their glucose regularly will see a huge reduction in their glucose levels when they use the 3x1 diet.

Be careful that you don't stuff yourself with breaded foods. Breaded meats for example are covered in flour, in other words, bread. If you order breaded shrimps you have to take into account that the breading on the shrimp is a Type F food and counts as a portion. You have to take into consideration the breading as a Type F food if you don't want to break your 2x1 or 3x1 Diet. You also shouldn't kid yourself by ignoring the VOLUME (space that they take up) of the foods. If you got an extra-large portion of fried potatoes and they, when spread out, take about ⅔ of the plate you should consider them 2 portions of F foods when taking into account their VOLUME. You have to use your common sense for this diet to work and not kid yourself.

In the case of a tasty baked potato, what I do is divide it in two, and eat half along with a nice salad and some meat. That way, I don't have to suffer from denying myself something and I don't break my 2x1 Diet. Naturally, if I am going to have a baked potato, I already know that I have to avoid the slice of bread that I always love to have. At times, what I do is order an appetizer that is high in protein, like a shrimp or seafood cocktail, oysters or even cheese and I ask the waiter not to bring any bread so that I'm not tempted.

With sandwiches and hamburgers the problem is that the majority of them, by proportion, and by VOLUME, are mostly bread. A hamburger, when you look at it on a plate and place the two pieces of bread in the proportions that they actually occupy on the plate, it looks like this:

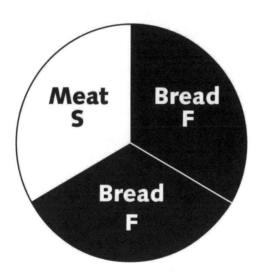

The amount of salad that they put on a hamburger is so small in comparison with the bread that you can't even consider it as your portion of Type S food. Sandwiches and hamburgers are not going to help you slim down because the bread that they contain produces too much insulin. That's why fast food restaurants have had such a negative impact on the general health of the population. As if these foods, that are high in refined carbohydrates like bread, weren't doing enough damage, fast food restaurants offer these hamburgers as combination meal promotions or "combo meals" with French fries (Type F) and soda (Type F).

Within the group of foods that are considered refined carbohydrates, like bread, there are different levels of quality. The reality is that white bread is digested very quickly. This allows your body to turn it into glucose very easily and later quickly into fat. You can always choose a whole wheat bread that is high in fiber and that will make it easier to boost your metabolism and slim down. That's why a sandwich is always less damaging when it is eaten with whole wheat bread as opposed to white bread. Bread, whether it is wheat or white, continues being a Type F by the amount of insulin production that it provokes in your body. But, if you have the opportunity to choose whole wheat bread over white, you will have more points in your favor.

On the subject of fruit, I can say that if the fruit has a sweet taste, this indicates that it is also high in carbohydrates and is a Type F food that makes us fat and it must be controlled. Fruits that are very sweet like bananas, mangoes, melons, pineapples and oranges, are all Type F foods. However, there are fruits that are not so sweet, like strawberries and apples that are considered Type S that make you slim down. In general, if the fruit is sweet it is a Type F food and if it isn't very sweet it is Type S.

If your situation has gotten to the point where you are very overweight or obese, think about it and you'll realize that you have been eating 5 to 8 times more of Type F foods (fattening) than foods that are Type S (slimming).

A dinner that starts with a slice of garlic bread and continues on to an appetizer of corn fritters and then to a 12 ounce steak with a large baked potato, along with corn on the cob, that you have with a Coca-Cola and finish off with a sugary dessert (cheesecake, ice cream), is like a 1x6 proportion between Type S foods and Type F foods. This would be disastrous for your metabolism.

So, choose a 2x1 or 3x1 Diet according to what you need and what your goals are at the time. You can also start with the 3x1 diet so that you can get results that motivate you or even achieve your goal first and, later, use the 2x1 Diet as a diet to stay slim. Whatever you choose to do, if you lower your consumption of Type F foods and increase your Type S foods you will see your fat disappear and your metabolism increase.

In the Diet 2x1 or Diet 3x1 there is no type of food that is prohibited. All types of food are acceptable and therefore you do not have to restrain yourself from anything. It's just a matter of reducing the proportion of Type F foods (fattening) so that they are never more than ⅓ of what you are going to consume if you are doing the 2x1 Diet. Or reduce the Type F to no more than ¼ of what you will consume if you are doing the 3x1 Diet. But, nothing is forbidden because the 2x1 and 3x1 diets are more a "lifestyle" than just diets.

The 2x1 combinations are endless. Here are a few that you might enjoy:

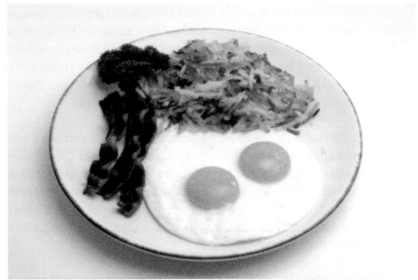

A 2x1 BREAKFAST: EGGS, BACON AND POTATOES

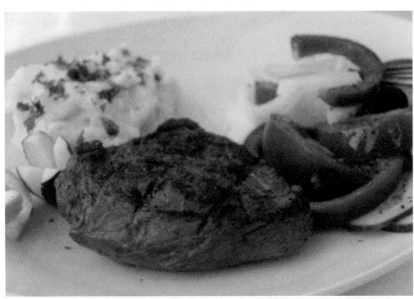

A 2x1 LUNCH OR DINNER: MEAT, SALAD AND MASHED POTATOES

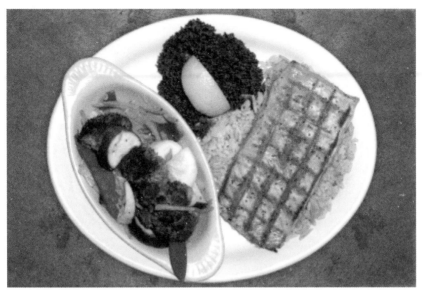

A 2x1 GRILLED SALMON OVER RICE WITH VEGETABLES

How To Survive "On The Street"

In order to guarantee success using the 2x1 and 3x1 Diets, it is good to have strategies or "tricks" that let us survive well while eating the food that is available "on the street"; in other words, cafeterias, restaurants and fast food restaurants.

Ideally, you would avoid fast food restaurants all together, but I realize that sometimes we don't have any other choice. It is good to know what to do when circumstances force us to eat what is closest to us even though it isn't the healthiest option.

It is to our benefit to become curious and learn what food combinations we can make with what's available in our environment. Typical lunch cafeterias usually have some meat dish, with some starch (potatoes, bread) and some salad or vegetables. This can be utilized to adjust it to our 2x1 or 3x1 diets.

For example, sometimes for lunch I order a sirloin steak with a baked potato and salad. When I go to eat I make sure that the amount of baked potato (Type F) that I eat isn't more than ⅓ of what I am going to eat in total. This generally means that I will eat approximately half of the baked potato on my plate. And of course, I drink water with my meal. Soft drinks, even diet ones, are fattening. (See the topic: DEHYDRATION)

Some fast food restaurants offer low carbohydrate options. Yet, all fast food restaurants, including McDonalds and Burger King, have salads with chicken breast. If I don't want salad I order other combinations but never accept their "combo offers" because they always come with some sort of side order that is high in carbohydrates (French fries, larger soft drink, corn bread) and very little protein (meat). For example, if I go to a KFC (*Kentucky Fried Chicken*), I order 2 chicken breasts, coleslaw salad and a bottle of water. Since the chicken breast is breaded I consider the crust as my portion of the Type F food. Therefore, I end up with a 2x1 made up of chicken (Type S), coleslaw (Type S) and the breaded crust (Type F); in the end, a 2x1.

The 2x1 of breaded chicken breast with coleslaw salad would look something like this:

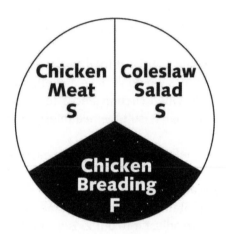

Subway has had brilliant marketing strategy: they make people think that they can lose weight while eating their low-fat sandwiches. They make people think that somehow their sandwiches, which are mostly bread (an F Type Food) won't make you fat as if your body knew the difference from their bread and others. It's all a lie.

Denny's, Cracker Barrel or any other diner in your area that is open 24 hours offers omelets, steaks, hash brown potatoes, grits, pancakes, French toast, sausages, waffles with blue berries and whipped cream. Out of these only the omelets or steaks will help you compose a 2x1 Diet plate.

I love spare ribs, but I know I can't eat them all the time, so I put a limit on how often I can eat them to once a week. When I order them I also order fried potatoes and I only eat half of them, and I also eat some sort of salad with lettuce and tomato, or some other combination. This keeps with the portions in my 2x1 Diet.

At times I order a grilled steak, French fries, and a Caesar salad. I make sure to eat only half of the French fries so that I don't go over my portion of Type F foods and again have a 2x1.

At my favorite Italian restaurant, the specialty, of course, is pasta. Pasta is high in carbohydrates and is a Type F food because it causes a huge reaction of insulin. Even so, I don't have to deny myself of it. What I do is order a main dish of beef (Type S) or fish (Type S) along with pasta (Type F) and my favorite sauce. I make sure that the amount of pasta (Type F) that I eat isn't more than ⅓ of what I eat in total. This could also work with 2 portions of beef or fish for every portion of pasta so that I don't break my 2x1.

When I go to steak restaurants I don't have problems with ordering food. They have shrimp cocktails (Type S) as an appetizer and I can order a nice steak with a portion of mashed potatoes or French fries that doesn't go over the ⅓ of what I eat in total. Steak restaurants sometimes also have pasta combinations (Type F) that are acceptable when the portion of pasta doesn't exceed ⅓ of what you eat in total.

European restaurants (French, German) offer good choices to combine a 2x1 Diet. The European eating custom (hard bread, little sweets and very little sugar) and the fact that they eat foods high in proteins (meat, cheese, ham, sausage) and a lot of salad and vegetables makes their food quite acceptable for our purposes. Fast food restaurants haven't had a huge growth or influence in Europe.

If I go to a Chinese restaurant I order different types of meals, avoiding those that have sweet sauces so as to avoid the sugar that they have in them. I order white rice to go with them and limit the portion of rice. The Chinese have a great variety of meals that are meat, seafood or poultry combined with stir-fried vegetables. All of these are acceptable for a 2x1 or 3x1 diet. It's a question of avoiding those that are too sweet like sweet-and-sour pork or chicken, which are cooked with a lot of sugar.

At Mexican restaurants I order "carnitas" (small pork pieces) and make sure that I don't go over by having too many corn or flour tortillas. The cheese dip is okay if I don't have too many of the tortilla chips that come with it. My favorite is a kind of taco that doesn't contain any flour. It has an outer tortilla made out of toasted cheese. This one is called a "pionero taco". There is another dish called "alambre gratinado" (meat and cheese). This is a dish made with pieces of chicken or beef that have been sautéed with onions, peppers, tomatoes and lots of white cheese. The "alambre gratinado" is served with flour tortillas, which I don't eat because the dish alone is a complete meal. Whatever the circumstance, I try to keep close to my 2x1 Diet without denying myself anything.

When someone becomes aware that it is the insulin hormone that produces fat in your body, they start to get creative in avoiding and lowering their consumption of those foods that force their body to produce a lot of insulin. It is a question of knowing that the following foods are Type F (fattening foods) because they cause a high production of insulin.

- Bread
- Cereals
- Chocolates
- Cooked beans
- Corn
- Flour
- Grits
- Milk

- Pasta
- Potatoes
- Rice
- Soft drinks
- Sugar
- Sweet fruits
- Sweets, candy
- Yams

Lowering your consumption of these foods can seem pretty tough at first for two reasons: 1) they are the most common foods in our diets, and 2) carbohydrates have a certain "addictive" power over us (see the topic CARBOHYDRATES ARE ADDICTIVE).

However, in reducing them, our anxiety and desire to eat them will disappear. If this topic causes you a certain amount of anxiety you will need the help that I suggest under the subject titled "BREAKING THE HABIT" that is covered later on in the book.

The reality is that when we increase our consumption of proteins (Type S foods), we decrease our hunger and the anxiety disappears. It is refined carbohydrates that cause the anxiety and the lack of control that comes with it. This is something that can be proven in starting a 2x1 or 3x1 Diet. In a couple of days, you will feel serene and without "cravings". In other words, you will have taken control of your body and your hormonal system.

If it happens that you are one of those people who don't like salads or vegetables, there is still a solution for you. The solution is to make sure that the PROPORTION of foods that you eat is always 2 portions of Type S foods (meat, fish, seafood, cheese, eggs) for every one portion of Type F foods (bread, pasta, flour, rice, etc.)

To successfully come up with a 2x1 or 3x1 PROPORTION you can make it even if you only eat two different foods. You can do this by increasing the proportion of the Type S (SLIMMING) while decreasing the proportion of the Type F (FATTENING). An example of this would be a breakfast of 2 fried eggs with a slice of toast.

Having only 2 foods you can see how you would end up with a breakfast of 2 eggs with one (1) slice of bread:

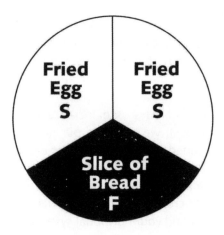

In the example above, you get the proportions of the 2x1 Diet using only 2 foods. The example also could have been of a lunch made up of larger amount of steak and onions (Type S) and lesser amount of fried potatoes (Type F). A large steak with half a portion of French fries does the trick of having a 2x1 Diet while using only 2 kinds of foods (steak and French fries). When you make sure that no more than ⅓ of your diet is of fattening foods (Type F) you will be able to slim down because you will be reducing the production of insulin in your body.

In other words, it's only a question of getting your consumption of those foods that produce a lot of insulin, Type F, to never be more than ⅓ of what you eat in total. This can be achieved even if you only eat 2 different foods. There are situations like eating a nice piece of barbequed meat and having it with a small corn on the cob. If the proportion of the meat that you eat is more or less double the proportion of the corn, you will have successfully created a proportion of 2x1.

In conclusion, we can survive "on the street" by using whatever we have available. The key is to know how to create the proportions that produce the least amount of insulin with the 2x1 or 3x1 diets.

"Diets" Don't Work

Different studies that have been done have revealed that approximately 95% of people that start a diet lose weight and then gain the weight back again in less than one year. This is saying that 95% of diets are failures. What good is it to suffer through a diet if very shortly after you've lost the weight you gain it all back again? What's the point in keeping yourself from eating the foods that you love if you're just going to gain back the weight you lost? What a miserable way of wasting time!

In reality, "diets" don't work. The traditional concept of "a diet" is the concept of "denying myself something" or "not allowing myself to eat something". It is a negative concept.

There is a human characteristic that sabotages all diets. It is the tendency to desire that which we are told we cannot have. Diabetics are told that they can't eat sweets, so what the diabetic person really wants to eat then, are sweets. The basic principal behind this human reaction seems to be that the "scarcity" always causes the "necessity".

The only real freedom that exists is the freedom of "being able to have" or "not being able to have" something. For example, an alcoholic "has to have" alcohol, and that is why he is an alcoholic. If he could "have it" or "not have it" he would simply be free to decide if he wanted the alcohol or not and wouldn't be an alcoholic. Whenever there is a situation where "I can't have" a certain substance, that creates a scarcity of it, and therefore, a necessity. It's a trap.

"Diets", generally speaking, are a type of "I can't have" and cause scarcities of substances and therefore create a feeling of necessity. I've been working for 20 years with thousands of people that have been slimming down. I constantly have to convince people that they don't have to deny themselves of any foods. I know from experience that if you start to deny yourself a piece of pie that you really want, you will eventually lose control and you will eat double or triple what you initially felt like eating.

People are accustomed to going, for example, to a nutritionist that asks them not to eat fat, or use salt, or eat sweets or some other prohibition. In other words, they get used to thinking in terms of "what I can eat and what I can't eat". That's why they fail; they deny themselves of the things that they really like. This is what makes them consider their diet to be an "enemy" because their "diet" denies them of the things that they really enjoy. The mind works by association. All of those things that block us from the pleasures of life could be considered our "enemies". The word "diet" has come to have a very negative connotation because it stands for "I can't have this, or I can't have that".

What I have seen that works is avoiding this limited concept of "a diet" and adopting the wide concept of what we call a "lifestyle". A "lifestyle" is a route that one freely chooses. If I know that certain foods cause serious harm when I eat them, it would be really irresponsible on my part to eat them excessively. That's not to say that I have to completely eliminate them forever as if my religion didn't allow it. What is optimum in life is to find a "balance". All extremes complicate life and make it more difficult to enjoy it.

The main goal of this book, *"The Power of Your Metabolism"*, is to create awareness. Don't deny yourself of anything or put yourself on a "diet". The idea is to understand which factors are the ones that speed up your metabolism and which are the ones that slow it down. The idea is to invite you to take part in a "lifestyle" where you eat all of the foods that you love responsibly, but with complete consciousness of the effect that each one of them has on your metabolism and health.

There aren't any foods that are bad for you. There are foods that can be very harmful to your metabolism and health if you eat too much of them. There isn't anything bad about a piece of pie. There isn't anything wrong with potatoes, bread, fried food, sweets, chocolates or any other kind of food. It is all a question of proportions and balance between them. You can enjoy EVERYTHING without abusing those that cause a lot of damage to your health like refined carbohydrates.

So, I'm inviting you to take part of a healthy "lifestyle" where you will feel much more energetic. Every day you will feel healthier and need medications less. It's a "lifestyle" that protects your metabolism and doesn't make you overweight or obese. Forget about the idea that it is a "diet". "Diets" don't work, "Lifestyles" do.

ON THE NEED FOR SNACKS

One of the most common recommendations that different experts tell people that want to slim down is to try to eat several small meals or snacks throughout the day. The logic behind this recommendation is that the body reacts by increasing the metabolism in response to eating the food and by having several small snacks the metabolism is increased. It sounds logical at first.

Did you know that just thinking about food increases the insulin levels in your blood and the hormones that cause hunger? This has been scientifically proven with laboratory analysis where they measure the different hormone levels in the blood of a group of volunteers before and after they had been thinking about food. Remember that your mind controls EVERYTHING. In thinking about your favorite dessert, you will have caused a reaction of insulin in your body.

Insulin is the hormone that makes you gain fat. It is a hormone that works as a "shopping cart" to take glucose to your cells. Without glucose and without the help of insulin, you simply can't get fat. Therefore, one of the main goals of the 2x1 and 3x1 Diet is to DECREASE the production of insulin in your body. In order to slim down, you must decrease the production of insulin to stop the accumulation of new fats, while you break the fats that you have already built up in your body.

Well, the reality is that if you really needed to have 5 or 6 meals or snacks during the day, your metabolism would have already passed the point of being able to be repaired or improved. Eating 5 or 6 small meals or snacks every day can initially cause weight loss, but it will be destroying the little metabolism that is left. Even low-calorie snacks increase the production of insulin and therefore the body never starts to use the hormone that has the opposite effect to insulin that is called *glucagon*[25]. When the blood glucose levels drop down, like what happens with the 2x1 or 3x1 Diets, instead of producing insulin, your body produces *glucagon*. This hormone, *glucagon*, turns your body fat into glucose again so that the body has food for its cells. In other words, it is the *glucagon* hormone that helps you slim down while insulin makes you fat. Having several small meals and snacks creates a situation where your body produces too little *glucagon* and thus it never really starts burning fat.

You see, all of the excess fat in your body was at one time, glucose, and the insulin turned it into fat. The sequence and formula is: "glucose + insulin = fat". *Glucagon* does the exact opposite of what insulin does. *Glucagon* breaks the fat down and turns it into glucose again. This is what makes you slim down and decrease your clothing size or waistline.

It is only by increasing the time between your meals that you will be able to slim down. The human body isn't designed to function like cattle that spend the day eating grass, or chickens that never stop eating corn. Having many meals, a day will stop your metabolism. You need three good meals a day that are high in protein and low in refined carbohydrates, and nothing more.

What always happens when someone does a 2x1 or 3x1 Diet is their hunger disappears! Yes, the 2x1 or 3x1 keeps hunger away for hours, to the point where sometimes you will find it difficult to eat lunch because you had such a good breakfast high in proteins. Many times, your body won't have the desire for more food even after 4 or more hours have passed since you had breakfast.

---

[25] Glucagon - It is a hormone produced by the pancreas and it is released when the glucose level in the blood is low (hypoglycemia). The action of glucagon is the opposite of insulin in that it breaks up fat and converts it to glucose.

The 2x1 Diet reduces your insulin levels (insulin causes hunger) and increases *glucagon* levels (*glucagon* gets rid of hunger). That's why you won't have to control your hunger for hours on end because it is impossible to be hungry if your body isn't producing very much insulin.

The recommendation of "having several snacks" or small meals a day originated from bodybuilders and diabetics. Bodybuilders and diabetics have special needs and are not the case of the common person. Bodybuilders lift weights and, in the process, consume a large amount of glucose. Therefore, they have to replace this glucose with small meals throughout the day.

In the case of diabetics, nutritionists have found that their glucose levels are unstable; in other words, too high (diabetes) or too low (hypoglycemia). The nutritionists' solution was "have several small meals or snacks throughout the day" to maintain their glucose levels. In my opinion and based on more than 8,000 diabetics that I have worked with on the NaturalSlim system, making diabetics eat every 2 to 3 hours was the wrong solution. In fact, it was the solution that made them the most overweight. It's the solution that guarantees you will always have high glucose levels and increased necessities for insulin.

Working with thousands of diabetics, we realized that their problem was with refined carbohydrates. Period. Nothing else caused more problems for diabetics than refined carbohydrates. When a person with diabetes does a 2x1 Diet or ideally a 3x1 Diet they will see their blood glucose levels stay stable for at least 4 hours after a meal that is high in proteins and low in refined carbohydrates. This is something that diabetic people can test with their blood glucose-testing device; it isn't just a theory.

Diabetics are the people that benefit most from the 2x1 or 3x1 Diets. In doing a 2x1 or 3x1 diet, they will feel a considerable increase of energy and their hunger will disappear. If they inject themselves with insulin, they will have to reduce the insulin dose in coordination with their doctor when doing the 2x1 or 3x1 Diet. This is something that always happens to diabetics that do the 2x1 Diet and especially those that follow the 3x1. These diets lower their body's needs for insulin.

Various scientific studies have found a correlation between the number of meals you eat a day and obesity. One study found that obese women, in general, eat one more meal a day than women who are not obese. It also found that overweight women tend to eat more snacks in-between their meals than women who are not overweight.

Naturally, the body needs an adaptation or adjustment period. If you start a 2x1 or 3x1 diet and you still feel the desire or need to have a snack don't let your body, go hungry. If you let yourself go hungry, your body will become stressed and that will cause the production of the stress hormone *cortisol,* which will make you gain fat. Therefore, never let your body feels hungry if you want to improve your metabolism and slim down. If you are still feeling a little hungry in-between your 3 main meals of the day, the solution is to have a snack that is high in proteins and low in refined carbohydrates.

The snacks that are going to make you slim down are foods like almonds, nuts, cheese, ham, or any other food that is low in carbohydrates. You can even have pork rinds for a snack. Remember that pork rinds have a lot of fat, but your body can't use this fat unless insulin is produced. If you don't eat refined carbohydrates for your snack, your body won't produce much insulin and it won't be able to use the fat from the snack to make you fatter. Your body can create new fat only with the help of insulin.

When people don't know this, they make the mistake of having a snack of cake, toast, cookies or some other food that is high in refined carbohydrates. These same things are what cause the increase of glucose and the insulin that causes more hunger.

No, you don't need to eat all day like a cow or a chicken. You don't need "snacks" if you do things right and understand how your body works. You will live free from the hunger that torments people with a slow metabolism.

MAXIMUM ACCELERATION

At times we find it necessary to slim down at a faster rate. It could be due to an upcoming wedding, a high school reunion or some other situation that puts pressure on us to slim down in a short amount of time.

There is a very quick and healthy way to slim down. The basic guidelines are:

- Follow the 3x1 Diet (very little refined carbohydrates)
- Have whey protein shakes for breakfast
- Add organic coconut oil to the shake
- Drink a lot of water
- Take high potency vitamins daily
- Eat mainly fish for protein
- Eat salad with every lunch and dinner
- Drink vegetable juice every evening
- Don't eat: soy, wheat, corn or pork
- Do exercise, like walking, 3-4 times a week

For breakfast, drink a whey protein shake with the organic coconut oil. This boosts your metabolism very efficiently.

During the "speeding up" process, follow a 3x1 diet (very little refined carbohydrates), in which the main protein is fish. Of all proteins, fish is the lowest in saturated fat and contains elements of vitamins and minerals that are essential to the functioning of the thyroid (iodine, selenium, omega 3 oils). In doing the speeding up diet, you should combine your fish with a good amount of salad and vegetables. You can have small amounts of refined carbohydrates like rice, potatoes, etc., but no wheat products (bread, pasta, bread crumbs, and flour, etc.).

If you don't like fish, which is really the best protein to have, you can use white meats (chicken, turkey). Fish is best because it is easy to digest and really does help you to slim down. Among fishing communities, obesity doesn't exist. No other protein is cleaner or easier to digest than fish meat. In addition, fish also contains natural oils called "omega 3", which are oils that "burn fat" and reduce cholesterol.

To slim down as quickly as possible, it helps to add vegetable juices to your diet every evening. There are various juicing machines for fruits and vegetables on the market that aren't too expensive. *Jack Lalanne* is a well- priced brand of juicers that you can get at stores like *Macy's* or *JC Penney's*. Canned or bottled vegetable juices like V8 vegetable juice will never give you the incredible results that you can obtain by juicing your own fresh vegetables.

The idea is to drink vegetable juices, not fruits. Vegetables are low in carbohydrates and provide minerals and nutrients that speed up your metabolism. With the juicer you can extract a mix of carrot, cucumber, radish, celery, broccoli, watercress and spinach juices, and then add a little bit of ginger and parsley for zest. You can have the vegetable juice mixture for dinner in the evening. It's amazing how the vegetable juices contribute to accelerating the process of slimming down. It's almost as if your body deflates when you drink these juices.

Vegetable juices could be considered near "miracles". For people who have high blood pressure, these juices tend to lower blood pressure. Fresh vegetable juices contain high amounts of potassium, which works as a diuretic and lowers blood pressure. Potassium is a mineral that counteracts the salt (sodium) in your body. In other words, when you consume potassium, your body passes any built-up salt (sodium) through your urine, which lowers your blood pressure.

You can use these vegetable juices as replacements for your dinner in the evening. They taste good and produce remarkable results. You can get the average juice extractor for less than $100 and it is a good investment for your health and metabolism.

The "maximum acceleration" diet is a technique that works for when you want to slim down quickly without compromising your health and going hungry.

If you like fish and you want to slim down very quickly, follow this "maximum acceleration" diet for a week and you will see the results. In my case, I use it to compensate for the damage that I've done from my little "slip-ups" during the weekend.

BREAKING THE HABIT

A s we saw before, refined carbohydrates have the power of causing an addiction. The addiction can be a light one (the minority of the cases), but in some cases it is a very strong addiction (the majority of the cases). There are people that are seriously "trapped" in this addiction and can't even go one day without their "fix".

I've seen cases where people must have their *Coca-Cola, Pepsi-Cola®, 7-Up®*, chocolate, candy, bread or some other refined carbohydrate every day. They simply <u>have to have them,</u> or they feel like something is missing. These people are hostages of their addiction to refined carbohydrates. If they try not to eat them, they feel very anxious and it affects their mood in a negative way.

If you feel anxious or have a strong "craving" for a certain food on a daily basis, be assured that what you are experiencing is an addictive relationship with this food. In my case, I had an addiction to rice, as I live in Puerto Rico where rice is a staple food. I thought that eating a meal without rice was like not eating at all. Believe me, rice was what caused my weight problem and my slow metabolism. There are other people whose addiction is to bread or cake, for some it is candy, and for many others, their addiction is to soft drinks like Coca-Cola. However, there are some that don't discriminate, and their addiction is to all refined carbohydrates in general, without caring what it might be.

To free yourself from one of these addictions it is important that you know two things:

1. That you should break away from your addiction GRADUALLY.

2. That you can experience unpleasant physical reactions. Drug addicts refer to them as "withdrawal symptoms".

If you feel that you are experiencing an addiction to a food, the first thing to do is to recognize that you have the addiction. The second is to come up with a plan to break away from the addiction. This plan should include having a day in which you can still have the food (rice, bread, chocolate, sugar, etc.), but a smaller amount than usual. This "preparatory" day, which is the day before breaking away from the food or the foods that are causing your addiction, is vital. The idea is to do it GRADUALLY, without causing a crisis in your body.

Starting on the "preparatory" day, or the day before completely breaking away from the addiction, you should begin drinking large quantities of water. The water hydrates your body and creates an environment that allows you to get rid of what your body wants to get rid of during the process. It is vital to drink as much water as you can.

The day that you totally break away should be a day in which you only eat meat (ideally chicken, turkey or fish), cheese (any kind), and eggs (fried, boiled, in an omelet or scrambled). There are only 3 types of foods that you should eat during that breaking away day: meat, cheese and eggs. For example, an omelet with cheese and sausages would be appropriate. It is pure protein and no carbohydrates.

During the breaking away day what you are trying to do is "break the habit" by getting rid of ALL the sources of carbohydrates in your body so that you can break your addictive relationship with them.

That's why during the break away day you aren't to eat any type of carbohydrates. This means that during that day, you won't even eat salad, vegetables, fruit or vegetable juices, milk, or have sugar in your coffee (you can have your coffee black) or eat anything that contains carbohydrates. You will eat only meat, cheese and eggs. You can eat all that you want of these three types of foods, and you won't feel hungry. Meats can be fried in oil, baked or cooked in some other way. You can use any condiments like garlic, oregano, etc. The way you prepare the meat doesn't matter, what you need to do is "break the habit", and you can achieve this by completely breaking away from all carbohydrates for one full day. The ideal scene is to do this for two full days and that way you will be sure that the addiction is broken for good.

During the breaking away period, drinking more water will be even more vital. Your body produces the hormone *cortisol* during the breaking away because taking away your addictive foods causes a certain level of stress. *Cortisol* is called "the stress hormone". The breaking away period causes stress to your body and water helps to remove this hormone while calming down your hormonal system.

If, in doing this, you experience reactions like migraines, headaches, itchy skin, vaginal discharge, diarrhea or muscle pain, then the problem is that your body is severely infected by the *candida albicans* yeast (see the topic *CANDIDA ALBICANS*, THE SILENT EPIDEMIC).

When your body is extremely infected by this yeast, which is what happens to many people who are overweight, the reaction to breaking away from carbohydrates can be very unpleasant. If it happens that the infection of the *candida* yeast is an extensive one, it can be made up of several million yeast organisms. This yeast completely depends on carbohydrates for its livelihood. Without carbohydrates, the yeast can't survive. This is why the yeast starts to die and rot inside your body when you break away from all carbohydrates in your diet; the yeast is left without its food. When this yeast starts to rot, it fills your body full of acids and toxins that the rotting yeast produces and causes all of the unpleasant symptoms like migraines, headaches, muscular pain and various others. Generally, the symptoms don't last more than a day, but I must say that they can be extremely unpleasant.

Within the NaturalSlim system, we've spent nearly 20 years helping thousands of people to break their addiction to carbohydrates. We have developed natural supplements that dramatically reduce the side effects of the withdrawal syndrome. At NaturalSlim, we also use special natural programs to cleanse the body of the *candida albicans* yeast, so that you can speed up your metabolism.

My reason for explaining the existence of these addictions is so as not to leave you with incomplete information. The ideal situation would be that a person that feels "addicted" to a food or a certain group of foods could receive the personalized attention of a system like NaturalSlim. This isn't always possible due to distance or other reasons. However, you should know that these addictions are a factor by which many people start their diet every Monday and by Wednesday they have already abandoned their diet and are eating "the same as always".

How To "Cheat" Intelligently

I n order to be successful in your goal of boosting your metabolism and slimming down, you should know which factors slow down and speed up your metabolism. This is what we have been talking about all along.

However, at times we find ourselves in social situations (parties, family celebrations, birthdays, etc.) where it is simply impossible or impractical to follow the 2x1 or 3x1 diet (see the topic A DIET YOU CAN LIVE WITH).

Well, there is no need to worry. If you find yourself forced to break your 2x1 or 3x1 Diet, what is important is that you know how to do it intelligently. The idea is to cause the least amount of damage as possible to your metabolism and to your goal of slimming down. There is a way to "cheat" intelligently.

Let's say you suddenly find yourself at a surprise birthday party for your best friend. There is a way that you can eat everything that is at the party but knowing how to do it. It is a question of avoiding major damage to what you have already accomplished by applying what you have learned so far.

In order, be able to eat everything in the party without causing major damage, you should first know how your body reacts to the foods that are high in carbohydrates. When you eat foods that are high in refined carbohydrates (cake, cookies, etc.), your body responds by producing a certain amount of insulin. The effect of the insulin is to lower the blood glucose levels that you have created by eating refined carbohydrates. The process goes something like this:

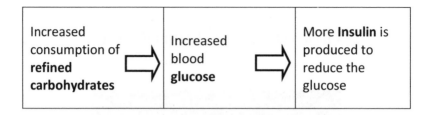

Increased consumption of **refined carbohydrates**	Increased blood **glucose**	More **Insulin** is produced to reduce the glucose

Doctors Rachael and Richard Heller wrote a book called *"The Carbohydrate Addicts Diet"*. They explain their discovery about how you can break your diet without causing much damage to your goal of slimming down.

These doctors discovered that your body learns from every one of the meals that you have. For example, if you have a breakfast high in carbohydrates, your body will have to produce enough insulin to manage the glucose that is created by the carbohydrates. For your next meal, lunch, your body will be expecting another meal high in carbohydrates and will be ready for a major production of insulin. In other words, your body is alive and learns how to "predict" what you are going to eat next. If, on the other hand, your breakfast is low in carbohydrates, your body will have to produce very little insulin and will be expecting a lunch that is also low in carbohydrates. Your body is learning, and it is you who are teaching it.

The other thing that the Heller doctors discovered is that when you eat carbohydrates your body always makes a first release of insulin, which is dependent upon what you ate in your previous meal. If you ate very little carbohydrates in your previous meal, the initial release of insulin in your body will be minor because your body has learned that you are eating very little carbohydrates. If on the contrary you ate a lot of carbohydrates at your previous meal your body will be ready to produce a large amount of initial release of insulin on your next meal.

The Heller's have also discovered that about an hour after you start eating, your body checks again to see how many carbohydrates you have eaten to see if it needs to produce more insulin. If your body senses that you have continued eating carbohydrates an hour later, then it will do a second release of insulin to be able to manage the additional glucose that will build up.

If you remember correctly, it is the action of insulin that makes us fat. The less insulin the body produces, the easier it will be for us to slim down. The more insulin is produced, the fatter we will get. Without insulin, it is impossible to get fat. The way to slim down is to decrease the production of insulin that your body makes in response to carbohydrates.

So, knowing this information about how your body works in response to what you eat, the Heller doctors taught us a way of "cheating" intelligently.

If you are going to break your diet and "cheat", the key is that you follow these 2 rules:

1. Never eat an excessive amount of refined carbohydrates if your previous meal was also high in carbohydrates. Your body will be waiting with a major release of insulin that will make you gain fat.

2. If you are going to eat a large amount of refined carbohydrates, make sure not to take longer than 1 hour to eat your meal. If more than an hour goes by from when you started eating carbohydrates, your body will produce a second release of insulin that will make you gain fat.

These are two rules that you have to follow to be able to "cheat" intelligently. If you follow these rules, you will be able to periodically, or when necessary, eat the amount of carbohydrates that the occasion requires without losing everything that you have accomplished up to that point.

Personally, if I know that I am going to a party in the evening, I try to be good during the day (breakfast and lunch) so that at the party that night I can indulge myself a bit and know that I'm not going to get fatter. Naturally, my indulging can't last more than 1 hour from start to finish. Therefore, when I'm going to eat, I eat. In other words, I don't stand around eating appetizers because I know that the time starts to count when I take the first bite and I want to avoid that second shot of insulin that the body produces if I continue eating for more than 1 hour.

You don't have to ever feel remorse or regret if you know what you are doing. You can "cheat", every once in a while, but do it intelligently.

THE TRUTH ABOUT CHOLESTEROL

After having read up to this point, it is possible that you are thinking that there is something wrong with all of this because I'm not asking you to cut back on fats and cholesterol. Instead, I'm telling you to eat butter, which has cholesterol, and to stop eating margarine, which has no cholesterol. These can sound like pretty weird ideas. However, you can understand the topic of cholesterol to the point where you won't ever have to worry about it again. Typically, those things that cause us the most problems are those that we don't totally understand.

I am aware of the fact that for more than 20 years the media has bombarded us with the dangers of cholesterol. The truth is that many times the media is more concerned with a type of sensationalistic reporting that sells them newspapers or increases their TV ratings, as opposed to actually informing the public of the facts. This is why the media isn't necessarily a good source of information about health topics; the information isn't always completely true. More often than not, pharmaceutical companies are hidden behind the news about our health. The pharmaceutical companies benefit from causing us enough fear to react by going to the doctor so that he or she can give us a prescription for their medications.

You surely have the ability to understand this subject of cholesterol and stop worrying about something that you can control on your own without any major problems or medications.

Cholesterol is a natural substance that your body produces, and it is essential to your health and life. All of your body cells, except the cells in your bones, contain cholesterol. We could say that cholesterol is a base material from which your body cells are constructed. Without cholesterol, cells couldn't be built.

This substance called "cholesterol" seems more like a type of wax than a fat. It is a substance that our body also uses to build our sexual hormones. For example, if you are a woman this is due to the fact that your body produces a lot of estrogen and only a little bit of testosterone. If you are a man, the opposite is true for you. Men have a lot of testosterone (masculine hormone) and little estrogen (female hormone). Your body makes these hormones by using cholesterol as a base material. Without cholesterol there wouldn't be sexual differences between us. Cholesterol is that important.

Years back, when the nation-wide campaign to "educate us" about cholesterol had just begun; we were told that all cholesterol was "bad". Then some years later it was discovered that there are 2 basic types of cholesterol: "bad" cholesterol and "good" cholesterol. The one called "bad" cholesterol is LDL (*"Low Density Lipoprotein"*). This "bad" cholesterol, LDL, is" low density" cholesterol, in other words, it is soft and gummy. Since it is soft it is also sticky, and it decomposes very easily. Imagine that the consistency of this "bad" cholesterol is like chewing gum. The problem is that it sticks to your arteries and decomposes, creating other toxic substances in your body.

On the other hand, there is the HDL cholesterol (*"High Density Lipoprotein"*) that they call the "good" cholesterol. This other type of cholesterol is tough, it doesn't decompose, and it doesn't stick. In fact, it is this "good" cholesterol, HDL, which gets rid of the "bad" cholesterol in your body, LDL. You can think of the "good" cholesterol, HDL, as having the tough consistency of a bowling ball.

There are other types of cholesterol like VLDL (*"Very Low Density Lipoprotein"*), but for our purposes here it is enough to know about only these two types, LDL the "bad" and HDL the "good" cholesterols.

The pharmaceutical industry has turned medications that control cholesterol into a gold mine. The statistics are clear; diagnoses of "high cholesterol" conditions are increasing each year that passes. Every year there are more people with "high cholesterol" and more people taking medications to control it. There are also many more cases of children and adolescents with high cholesterol.

All of this is happening while, each year that goes by, people consume less and less foods that contain cholesterol. In other words, in our days, supermarkets and food stores are full of products that are "cholesterol free". When a food is "cholesterol free", they prominently advertise it on the label because the manufacturers know that the public has a fear of cholesterol and uses it to their benefit to increase their sales. These "cholesterol free" products are also frequently advertised on T.V.

Butter is hardly eaten anymore in comparison with margarine. This happened due to the fact that margarine is sold as a "cholesterol free" alternative, since real butter has cholesterol.

The same thing happened with eggs. The consumption of eggs in the United States has gone down more than 40% in the last 30 years. This is again due to the massive campaign against cholesterol. From there were born new million-dollar industries and "cholesterol free" products like the egg substitute *Egg Beaters*. According to the advertisements, eggs contain cholesterol; therefore, we should either cut back on them, or stop eating them altogether.

All of this also brought about the production of polyunsaturated[26] oils like corn, vegetable and sunflower oil that have caught on quickly due to being "cholesterol free".

We have exchanged butter for margarine, pig fat (which was used for frying) for corn oil, and eggs for imitation eggs — all of this to switch to "cholesterol free" products. However, each year there

---

[26] Polyunsaturated oils can be found mostly in grain products, corn, soybeans and fish oil. They have been dubbed the "healthy oils" but there is nothing "healthy" about them.

are more and more people with high cholesterol! There are more people with clogged arteries from cholesterol and more young people having premature heart attacks. So, we eat much less cholesterol than before, yet we have more cholesterol running through our blood. This doesn't make any sense! It's like saying that the less money I deposit in my bank account, the more money I will have in it. How can we have more cholesterol in our body if we are consuming less of it?

Well, there is an explanation. We aren't going crazy yet. The reality is this:

OUR CHOLESTEROL GOES UP WHEN OUR CONSUMPTION OF REFINED CARBOHYDRATES GOES UP!

If you don't eat refined carbohydrates excessively, it is IMPOSSIBLE that you will have high levels of "bad" cholesterol. The only exception to this, is if you have a hypothyroid (low thyroid function) condition that hasn't been detected. A deficient thyroid always increases your cholesterol (see the topic on PROBLEMS WITH THE THYROID GLAND SYSTEM).

So, "high cholesterol" is equal to "excess of refined carbohydrates" or hypothyroidism. They have recently been blaming the "hereditary factor", but the reality is that it has never been scientifically proven.

The same reasons why our population is overweight and obese are the same reasons that cause the "high cholesterol" conditions. If you don't believe it, go to your doctor and take a cholesterol test. Later, start a 2x1 or 3x1 diet and see how your cholesterol goes back down to normal in 30 to 60 days. I've seen thousands of people who were overweight because they were addicted to carbohydrates. As soon as they started controlling their intake of refined carbohydrates, they started slimming down and their cholesterol, in ALL of the cases, went back to "normal". This happened even when they were eating butter with cholesterol, eggs with cholesterol and meat with cholesterol.

The human body has a sophisticated mechanism of controlling its cholesterol levels. When you eat meat which contains cholesterol, your body detects it and orders the liver to produce less cholesterol. If you avoid cholesterol in all of your foods, your body tells the liver to produce more cholesterol to compensate for the cholesterol that you aren't giving your body. Cholesterol is essential for your body and if you don't give it the cholesterol it needs, it will make it anyway. We can say that the body self-regulates itself unless it is forced to make more cholesterol because of excessive carbohydrate consumption or an undetected hypothyroid condition.

Now, we could say that cholesterol is a type of "building material". It is like the cement that we use to build houses. Cholesterol is the "cement" that the body uses to build the walls of the cells. That's why when you are getting fatter from eating an excess of refined carbohydrates and from a high production of insulin, your cholesterol is also going to go up. To be able to build new fat cells, your body needs a lot of new cholesterol. So, while you are getting fatter little by little, your cholesterol will continue increasing its availability in your body.

Everyone that does a diet that controls their intake of refined carbohydrates like the 2x1 or 3x1 Diet lowers their "bad" cholesterol, LDL, while increasing their "good" cholesterol, HDL.

Cholesterol is a "building material" not just for building new cells, but also to repair damaged cells. So, your body uses it to cover up flaws or breaks in areas where there are damaged cells. This is why people who have cancer have increased cholesterol levels. Cancer causes extensive cellular destruction and your body produces much more cholesterol than usual in an attempt to "repair" the cells that the cancer has been destroying.

If you enjoy a having spare ribs for dinner, don't worry about your cholesterol. Just be careful not to have your spare ribs with another food that is high in carbohydrates like mashed potatoes, especially if you are already suffering from high cholesterol. Refined carbohydrates are what raise your cholesterol. Salads and vegetables are natural carbohydrates that lower your cholesterol. In general, everything that increases the production of insulin in your body will raise your cholesterol levels. If you control your refined carbohydrates, your production of insulin will go down, as well as your cholesterol.

It could be that your doctor has told you the exact opposite of what I am telling you (I'm not a doctor). You can see it for yourself; do a lab test after doing the 2x1 or 3x1 diet for a while. You'll be surprised!

I have personally helped dozens of doctors that were overweight and had high cholesterol in bringing their cholesterol levels back down to normal. That was easy. The hard part was getting them away from the refined carbohydrates so that they could do it.

I can't blame the doctors for their lack of knowledge of the causes of high cholesterol. Believing that a person has high cholesterol because they eat an excess of foods that contain cholesterol sounds logical, but it is not correct. In general, doctors study nutrition for less than 12 hours, and the scientific study of the metabolism certainly isn't a subject in medical school. Add this to the massive propaganda that the doctors receive from pharmaceutical companies through their pharmaceutical sales representatives. You will see that the information that they receive has been put together so that they sell medications, not to get rid of the causes of high cholesterol. These simple, yet effective ideas of lowering the excess of refined carbohydrates in your diet to eliminate the CAUSE of high cholesterol are never going to be popular amongst pharmaceutical companies, but they are indeed the truth.

What you should know about eggs is that they are a perfect protein. Eggs don't have "bad" cholesterol, LDL, which is the one that sticks to your arteries. Eggs only contain "good" cholesterol, HDL. Eating eggs everyday can only lower your "bad" cholesterol. This information was the subject of the Times magazine cover page in July of 1999. I started researching it, testing it with thousands of NaturalSlim members, and found that it is definitely true. Eating eggs everyday lowers your "bad" cholesterol. Naturally, don't go and eat your eggs with a big piece of bread or some pancakes because you'll see that your "bad" cholesterol will go up.

Not too long ago, the University of California, School of Medicine did a study in which they had 1,934 men and women eat up to 14 eggs a week. Even though each egg had some 250 milligrams of cholesterol, the researchers were surprised when they didn't find any significant increase of cholesterol amongst the participants of the study. There have been other studies that have confirmed this. Even so, the news media hasn't released this information so that the public will stop avoiding eating eggs. This type of "positive" news that doesn't involve sensationalism, tragedy or danger simply isn't of interest to the news.

When you start a 2x1 or 3x1 Diet you might notice that your cholesterol levels will go up a little. Don't worry; it is natural for your cholesterol to go up a little because in doing the diet you will start to slim down. Slimming down breaks up a good amount of your fat cells and they release their cholesterol content into your blood. The cholesterol increase that you might notice in a lab test is also the same cholesterol that is leaving your body. Give it a little bit of time and you'll see that it will keep going down with every lab test that you do.

Even though we are talking about cholesterol, it is important that you know that the most dangerous substance for your heart is not cholesterol, but triglycerides[27]. Almost all of the publicity has been given to cholesterol because there is a variety of medications to lower cholesterol and this has created a huge potential market. However, what you should avoid is having high triglycerides because they are what are truly dangerous. High triglycerides mean that there is too much fat floating in your bloodstream. There is more likely a relation between high triglycerides and heart problems than a relation between high cholesterol and heart problems.

Luckily, nothing brings your triglyceride levels back to normal faster than lowering your intake of refined carbohydrates. A 2x1 or 3x1 Diet will bring your triglycerides back to normal in no time.

Cholesterol should never be a problem for you if you understand what causes high cholesterol levels and take control of what you eat and lower your consumption of refined carbohydrates. In doing so, you will have taken control of your cholesterol, as well as your triglycerides.

---

[27]Triglycerides - Triglycerides are fats. All fats and oils are triglycerides. They are called triglycerides because the molecules that make up all fats and oils always contain 3 (tri) extension lines made up of fatty acids hooked to a backbone of glycerin.

WE ARE ALL DIFFERENT

Research investigations are adventures that sometimes lead us down strange pathways and in the middle of this adventure I found myself studying the relation between cancer and diabetes. This time I was starting to investigate the subject of diabetes for the purpose of writing my new book, which I had decided to call *Problem-Free Diabetes*. It would seem that these two subjects, diabetes and cancer, are not related, but through the years I have learned to keep an open mind so that I can explore all the possibilities without my own judgments getting in the way about a subject. As the saying goes "There's none so blind as those who will not see"; this correctly applies to the field of investigations.

I cannot help from being extremely curious and I always try to take things from the stance of "you can always learn more about any subject". On the other hand, I recognize that in the past sometimes I've been wrong about an issue, and I have had to swallow my own words. It does not bother me to discover that I am wrong if at the end of the day I also manage to better understand the causes or solutions to a health problem.

Recently, I discovered that <u>I was wrong</u> pertaining to an important matter. My mistake was that, although the diet recommendations on the 2x1 and 3x1 Diet in this book have already produced "miraculous" results for thousands of people, people who managed to not only lose weight, but regain their health and even control their diabetes, there was a major factor that had not been made clear to readers: **we are not all the same!** What I mean is, everyone's body is different, with different hereditary factors and that which can makes it so that some food which often

233

may be good for some of us, could work like poison for others. Biochemical individuality definitely exists.

In the past, I had noticed that some individuals were obviously carnivores (meat eaters) while others were more inclined towards a vegetarian diet. I had no explanation for this other than it appeared to be something hereditary.

While studying the subject of cancer and its possible relationship to diabetes, I discovered the work of Dr. William Donald Kelley, a dentist who was heavily persecuted in the 80s because he was dedicated to curing cancer and who is said to have treated over hundreds of thousands of cases of cancer with his therapy based on protease enzymes (enzymes that digest proteins). I also studied the research conducted by Dr. Nicholas Gonzalez from New York who continues to offer and work on improving cancer treatments that originated from Dr. Kelley.

From the books and conferences I studied by Dr. Kelley and Dr. Gonzalez about cancer, I realized that there were undoubtedly significant differences between certain types of metabolisms, most of which had to do with the nervous system. Again, not all bodies are the same. I learned that while it is true that some people have been successful in reducing a cancerous tumor by adopting a vegetarian diet, there have also been cases where a vegetarian diet has had the opposite effect; that is, it would cause the cancerous tumor to grow. On the hand, there are also cases where the only thing that managed to reduce cancer progression was to adopt a carnivorous diet.

What Dr. Kelley and Dr. Gonzalez discovered in their respective anti-cancer practices was that there are several types of metabolisms, which vary depending on the type of nervous system that the person has. And that in fact there is no diet that is the perfect or ideal for everyone on the planet. There are ethnic groups predominantly composed of vegetarians, while there are others with an abundance of carnivores. This made me realize that even for those who seem to eat "everything", it is still found that certain foods, depending on the type of metabolism, tend to be better than others. When it comes to boosting the metabolism, it is important to know what types of foods should be favored for each individual type of diet. To figure this out, it is first necessary to discover what an individual's metabolism may favor: be more carnivore or to be more vegetarian.

It can easily be found throughout history that no diet can be a "one-fits-all" type of diet. For example, in the 60s the Dalai Lama, who is the spiritual leader of Tibetan Buddhism, had met an Indian man who was on a strict vegetarian diet. The Dalai Lama was so impressed by this man's diet that he too followed the same completely vegetarian diet. After two years of eating this way, he became ill with hepatitis. After trying several methods recommended by his doctor that ultimately did not work, his doctor then recommended that he start eating meat again, which finally helped him recover from the illness. For some reason the regimen of a strict vegetarian diet had reduced the Dalai Lama's body's defenses and rendered him ill. As soon as he began to eat meat again he started to feel better and his viral infection stopped, restoring health and energy that had been lost. The Dalai Lama, from that point on, continued to consume meat as part of his diet.

As an ethnic group, the Tibetan Buddhists had never had a history of a vegetarian diet. For one, it is very difficult to grow vegetables or grains in the dry and Rocky Mountains of the Himalayas where they lived. However, there are ethnic groups in India where vegetarianism is the norm and people become sick or weakened when they consume meat. Without a doubt, all human bodies are different.

For you to understand this and to benefit in terms of improving your metabolism and health, I will explain a little about the function of the body's nervous system. I will try to make this as simple as possible.

The functions of all organs (brain, heart, lungs, etc.) and glands (thyroid, pancreas and muscles of the body) are controlled via the autonomous nervous system. The autonomous nervous system consists of nerves that could be considered the control cables of the body, similar to the electrical wiring in a building. Although the majority of nerve impulses that control body functions happen unconsciously (without thinking or deciding about each one) some of the processes of the body, such as breathing, work in tandem with our conscious mind and can be affected by decisions and thoughts. The autonomous nervous system controls heart rate, digestion, respiration rate, salivation, perspiration, diameter of the pupils, urination or defecation and even sexual arousal.

This "wiring" (nervous system) that we call "autonomous nervous system" is itself divided into two systems that counteract each other. One of these two systems is the type of nervous system referred to as "sympathetic" (has nothing to do with being nice, by the way!) and the other nervous system is called "parasympathetic". The two parts of the autonomous nervous system, sympathetic and parasympathetic, work opposite to one another. In fact, they could be better said to be "complementary" to each other. They complement and even complete each other. The sympathetic nervous system could be compared to an accelerator of a car because, just like in a car, it will *accelerate* body movements. The parasympathetic system, on the other hand, could be compared to the brakes in a car because it will stop or inhibit the body's movements. The main actions of the sympathetic nervous system can be summarized as "fight or flight" as such actions require very fast and nervous excitement. For this reason, and to avoid using the medical term, which is harder to memorize, I have decided to call it an "EXCITED" nervous system. In contrast, the main actions of the parasympathetic nervous system could be summarized as "relax, rest and digest" because they are passive actions where excitement would be detrimental. To help you remember the information related to this type of nervous system I decide to call it the "PASSIVE" nervous system.

During the cancer treatments used by Dr. Kelly and Dr. Gonzalez in in their practice, it was discovered that some individuals had a nervous system that was predominantly "sympathetic", or as I call it, EXCITED. Others, were found to have a nervous system that was predominantly "parasympathetic" or as I call it, PASSIVE.

Those that have an EXCITED nervous system need certain foods to help soothe it (such as vegetables, green salads, light proteins like white meat or yogurt) and those of us with a PASSIVE nervous system need foods that excite the metabolism (such as red meat, solid protein like cheese and a greater amount of fat). The ideal state for any of us is a BALANCE between an EXCITED nervous system and a PASSIVE nervous system.

Dr. Kelley had ten different classifications for the nervous system. Five were predominantly EXCITED and the other five were predominantly PASSIVE. For example, the five types of the nervous systems that were classified as PASSIVE ranged from slightly passive to highly passive. In other words, there are degrees of both the EXCITED and PASSIVE types of nervous systems. For example, there are people with an EXCITED nervous system that can always seem to be "jumpy and nervous" and find it almost impossible to be sitting quietly (much like my wife who just cannot sit still!). Then, there are others, like me, who seem to be more like "thinkers" who have PASSIVE nervous system and find it difficult to even consider the idea of exercise.

In the ancient culture of China there is something called the "yin" and "yang". It refers to two conditions, which are contrary and counteract each other, yet also balance each other out. According to Chinese beliefs the "yin" is the PASSIVE state of rest and relaxation, whereas "yang" is the action or EXCITED state. It may be odd, but there seems to be some truth in the idea and popular belief that "opposites attract", as the Chinese "yin" and "yang" do. I have often observed that many couples tend to be composed of one PASSIVE and one EXCITED nervous system.

As my primary purpose is to educate people in improving their metabolism, health and conditions such as diabetes, I chose to use the terms PASSIVE nervous system and EXCITED nervous system because I realized that medical terms such as "sympathetic" and "parasympathetic" were not easy to memorize. I am only referring to the type of nervous system that is dominant in each person, and the terms PASSIVE or EXCITED have nothing to do with personality or the sexual activity of a person. One must know how to distinguish and differentiate between the body of a person and the personality, which is himself, not his body. The body does not have a "personality", nor does it have "opinions and attitudes" as people or a personality would. Sometimes we encounter people who seem to be "passive" due to their quiet and peaceful personality and yet still have a body with an EXCITED nervous system. The reverse is also true. So, you have to keep in mind that these classifications or types of nervous systems (PASSIVE or EXCITED) relate solely to what part of the nervous system is most dominant in your body. They have nothing to do with a person's personality, attitude or way of behaving.

In order to achieve higher energy levels and optimum health (as well as successful weight loss), it is vital to determine if one's nervous system is more inclined towards an EXCITED or PASSIVE nervous system. Knowing this, one can work towards developing the best possible balance of the two, which is the primary goal for improving your metabolism and health in the best way possible.

What I have observed in regard to either type of nervous system (EXCITED or PASSIVE) is that an individual's metabolism will react differently depending on the activity or inactivity of the nervous system. For example, nothing is more powerful in the human body than hormones, which are produced in response to the impulses of the nervous system. People whose nervous system is generally EXCITED tend to produce much more of the stress hormones, *adrenaline* and *cortisol*. Adrenaline, a hormone related to stress, forces the body to maintain high levels of glucose (also referred to as blood sugar) because its main function is to "tell" the liver to convert more of its glycogen (a form of glucose stored in your liver) into glucose. However, by increasing your glucose levels, your body will also produce a greater amount of insulin. As covered in previous chapters, high glucose levels will become fat when the hormone, insulin, is present.

On the other hand, when a nervous system is EXCITED, the stress hormone cortisol is also produced and this, in turn increases the levels of blood glucose that will create an accumulation of fat, especially in the abdomen. This is further explained in the chapter entitled *Stress Makes You Gain Weight.* Having an over-excited nervous system can affect the hormonal system and cause obesity; the nervous excitement stimulates the production of hormones like adrenaline, cortisol and insulin, all of which contribute to weight gain or difficulties in losing weight.

On the opposite hand, people who have a PASSIVE nervous system produce a greater amount of the neurotransmitter serotonin, which has a calming effect. A person with a PASSIVE nervous system has a much higher tendency to gain weight because their system is in a state of "rest, relaxation and accumulation". These are people with a "slow metabolism" who find it more difficult to lose weight and easily gain weight. Their entire nervous system is PASSIVE, which translates into very little movement. PASSIVE nervous systems, when excessively predominant in the body, can be found to create a condition of accumulated fat over the *entire* body.

In order to simplify this, we could say that in general there are two types of bodies and metabolisms, as follows:

1) An **EXCITED** nervous system for which the ideal diet would consist of primarily vegetables and salads, with small portions of lean protein (chicken, turkey, white fish), low in fat and salt.

2) A **PASSIVE** nervous system where it would be most beneficial to the individual to consume high-density concentrated protein (red

meats, cheese, and eggs). This type can tolerate a greater amount of fat and salt, because both can create stimulating effects on the body.

I had already noticed that my wife and I seemed to have our own distinct metabolisms and body types. She favors a diet rich in salads and vegetables to slim down, while for me it is impossible to lose weight if I do not consume enough red meat and fat in my diet. In fact, the times I tried to be a vegetarian I always felt physically weak and got sick, at least with the common cold. My wife, on the contrary, suffers indigestion from red meat and feels sick especially with pork, which is meat with a high fat content.

Theoretically speaking, there should be at least some individuals whose nervous system is in complete balance. I could also safely assume that individuals with a balanced nervous system, most likely do not suffer from obesity or diabetes. Diseases and problems with an individual's metabolism seem to be partly caused by a nervous system that is either too EXCITED or too PASSIVE. In other words, like everything in life, the extremes are what seem to hurt us.

The body's nervous system controls all the glands that produce hormones (including the thyroid, pancreas, ovaries, testes, adrenals, etc.). Hormones, in turn, control the production of energy in the body in addition to the creation or utilization of fat. The problems of the metabolism and health often originate with a hormone and it is logical to conclude that if the nervous system is too EXCITED or too PASSIVE, you might also have hormonal problems in addition to your metabolism problems. On top of that, hormonal imbalances can cause undesirable emotional states or what some would call "mental problems" or even depression. In short, the issue of a nervous system being too PASSIVE or too EXCITED can affect the way a person feels or behaves.

We also know that excessive stress causes a nervous reaction in the body that forces the adrenal glands to produce excess cortisol. We know that diabetics have problems with the production of the hormone insulin, which is produced by the pancreas. Some experts have said that Type II diabetes (non-insulin dependent), of which 90% of diabetics suffer from, is caused by severe stress conditions (such as a loss of a loved one, accidents, work or marital problems, etc.) all of which obviously can affect the nervous system. So, a nervous system that at one point becomes overly excited can cause damage to the glands that produce hormones and become the cause of diabetes or a condition of hypothyroidism.

Identifying your nervous system as EXCITED or PASSIVE should not be confused with having a "slow metabolism" or a "fast metabolism". We are referring here to the nervous system and what we want to know is what's the dominant trend of the nervous system, as it pertains to your body. As covered earlier, the nervous system carries signals that control glands within the body, which in turn produce hormones that control the overall processes and energy of the body. From this, it becomes obvious that <u>the state or condition of one's nervous system will be a determining factor on one's metabolism.</u>

EXCITED nervous systems will force the body to produce an excess of stimulants and stress hormones like adrenaline and cortisol. This inevitably has an effect on the metabolism. On the other hand, a PASSIVE nervous system will achieve higher production levels of calming hormones like serotonin; yet, a body with a PASSIVE nervous system will produce less of thyroid hormones that control energy production and the metabolism.

With PASSIVE nervous systems, the "slow metabolism" and conditions such as hypothyroidism are much more common. In principle, both the EXCITED nervous system as the PASSIVE nervous system can cause obesity because they are extreme conditions in which there is no balance, thus creating a hormonal disparity.

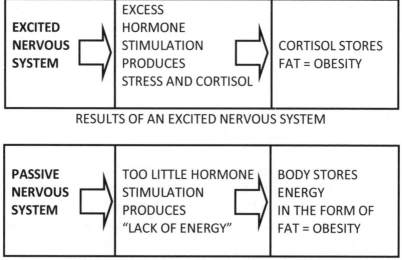

RESULTS OF AN EXCITED NERVOUS SYSTEM

RESULTS OF A PASSIVE NERVOUS SYSTEM

The advantage of knowing if your body is leaning more towards the EXCITED system or to the PASSIVE system is that it allows you to decide how to adapt and modify the 2x1 or 3x1 Diet for your particular body type. Adjusting your diet to the type of nervous system you have will help you feel more energetic and will simultaneously help you slim down, control diabetes and improve your overall health. To my understanding and based on what I have observed in hundreds of people, properly selecting your ideal food based on your type of nervous system (EXCITED or PASSIVE), will help you achieve your goals much faster and even leave you feeling better emotionally.

Note that the 2x1 or 3x1 Diet teaches you to portion out the F (fattening food) or S (slimming food) on your dish. But even within these two general types of food (fattening or slimming) there are even further choices between the two. Look below at the characteristics of each of these two types of nervous systems. Try locating which way your nervous system leans towards, whether it is towards the EXCITED or the PASSIVE side. This may be of some importance to you because by determining which way your body is inclined nervous system-wise you can then make better food choices. Remember, your body and what works best for it will not be the same as anyone else's.

Take a look at the next tables to determine which type of nervous system your body is inclined towards:

2 TYPES OF NERVOUS SYSTEMS BASED ON WHAT IS MORE DOMINANT	
EXCITED	**PASSIVE**
THESE ARE ALSO CALLED:	
SYMPATHETIC NERVOUS SYSTEM	PARASYMPATHETIC NERVOUS SYSTEM
"YANG" IN CHINA	"YIN" IN CHINA

Familiarizing yourself with the basic characteristics of both types of nervous systems (PASSIVE or EXCITED) will help you understand the most marked differences between the two. Later in the chapter you will be able to do a TEST TO DETERMINE YOUR NEROVOUS SYSTEM TYPE, which will allow you to determine if your nervous system is predominantly PASSIVE or is EXCITED. The purpose is to adjust the 2x1 or 3x1 Diet to fit your specific body type and thus improve the overall efficiency of your metabolism.

When an EXCITED nervous system is active, the body prepares for the physical act of "fight or flight" which limits your digestive capacity. Logic dictates that you cannot "fight or flight" when digesting. For example, if a person is quietly having dinner and someone brings very bad news or has to suddenly run because there's an emergency, your digestion will surely be negatively impacted. Here you can see how the EXCITED and PASSIVE nervous system reflect and influence your body's digestive system:

DIGESTIVE TENDENCIES:	
EXCITED	**PASSIVE**
DIGESTIVE SYSTEM WEAK OR DELICATE	EFFICIENT DIGESTION OF ANY FOOD
DOES NOT DO WELL WITH LATE NIGHT MEALS	CAN EAT ANYTIME OF THE DAY
CAN NOT TOLERATE SATURATED FAT	CAN TOLERATE SATURATED FAT

Once you know what your dominant type of nervous system is you will be able to better understand the functioning of your body's hormone system. This will help you better manage hormonal conditions such as diabetes or hypothyroidism. Also, you will now know the degree of importance that stress management might be for you.

Some hormonal characteristics that differ between the EXCITED nervous system and the PASSIVE system would be:

BASIC CHARACTERISTICS:	
EXCITED	**PASSIVE**
EXESSIVE ADRENALINE THAT EXCITES	THE CALMING SEROTONIN HORMONE DOMINATES
PANCREAS PRODUCES LITTLE INSULIN	PANCREAS PRODUCES TOO MUCH INSULINE
TENDENCY TOWARDS HYPERTHYRODISM	TENDENCY TOWARDS HYPOTHYRODISM

The following characteristics exist, which also help to differentiate between these two types of nervous systems:

OTHER BODY-RELATED CHARACTERISTICS:	
EXCITED	**PASSIVE**
RAPID PULSE	SLOWER PULSE
FASTER HEART RATE	SLOWER HEART RATE
TEND TO HAVE HIGH BLOOD PRESSURE	TEND TO HAVE LOW BLOOD PRESSURE
DIALATED PUPILS	CONSTRICTED PUPILS

When we speak of "a tendency" we mean a kind of inclination towards a certain state. However, when something has a "tendency" it just means that it has a high chance of happening. It's like when they survey the public before political elections and the survey results reflect "a tendency indicating that the candidate John Doe will win the elections." But when Election Day arrives, it is possible that John Doe does not turn out to be the winner because the tendency reflected in the surveys did not materialize. The "tendencies" are not absolutes and therefore can vary.

However, by knowing the trends and tendencies of each type of nervous system, EXCITED or PASSIVE, we can better understand the inclination of each type.

OTHER CHARACTERISTICS:	
EXCITED	**PASSIVE**
MUSCULAR PHYSIQUE	FLACCID PHYSIQUE
MORE INCLINED TOWARDS BEING PHYSICALLY ACTIVE	MORE INCLINED TOWARDS A SEDENTARY LIFESTYLE
TENDENCY TO HAVE CONSTIPATION	LITTLE TO NO PROBLEMS WITH CONSTIPATION
LESS PROBABILITY OF SUFFERING FROM ALLERGIES	GREATER PROBABILITY OF ASTHMA OR ALLERGIES
INSOMNIA OR DIFFICULTY WITH SLEEP	SLEEPS WELL

HAS A "SWEET TOOTH" OR IS A SUGAR ADDICT	LIKES SALTY FOODS, CONDIMENTS AND SPICES
LOVES COFFEE, WHICH WILL PROVIDE ENERGY AND EVEN "CLEAR" THE MIND	INTOLERANCE TO COFFEE, TOO MUCH COFFEE CAN CAUSE NERVOUSNESS

The 2x1 or 3x1 Diet will work best if you take these factors into account and choose the food you eat based on your type of nervous system. The 2x1 or 3x1 Diet determines the proportions between S-type (slimming) foods and F-type (fattening) foods, while your specific type of nervous system will determine the type of protein you should have (examples: high fat proteins, such as beef, pork, red fish, salmon, or tuna or low-fat proteins, such as chicken, turkey, white fish, low-fat cheeses, etc.). So, knowing your dominant type of nervous system lets you fine tune the selection of foods that make up your 2x1 or 3x1 Diet, so you can obtain the best possible results and thus, improve your metabolism. Food fuels your body just like gasoline fuels a car. Furthermore, just like there are cars that run on gasoline and others that run on diesel, there will be foods that are more appropriate for PASSIVE systems and some that are more appropriate for EXCITED systems.

For example, if your nervous system is the EXCTED type, eating plenty of vegetables and salads (which have a calming effect) will greatly benefit you. Additionally, fresh vegetable juices as covered in the chapter "Maximum Acceleration" are highly recommended. You can also include light proteins such as chicken, turkey and white fish (instead of salmon as it is high in fat) as (S) slimming type of food when you proportion your meals per the 2x1 or 3x1 Diet. Keep in mind that EXCITED nervous systems typically have trouble digesting proteins and fats properly, so you may need to assist your body with a digestive enzyme supplement.

If your nervous system turns out to be the PASSIVE type, you can consume more foods containing oils and fats, especially if you are careful not to overdo the consumption of F (fattening) Type

Foods. The F Type Foods are what force your body to produce more insulin. Insulin is the hormone that converts glucose into fat and allows the fats that you eat with your food to collect and ultimately get stored as body fat.

TEST TO DETERMINE YOUR TYPE OF NERVOUS SYSTEM

Well, you now have a general idea of the differences between the EXCITED and PASSIVE nervous systems. It is time to determine with a simple test, which is the more dominant nervous system in your body. The test consists of looking over 5 of the EXCITED nervous system indicators and marking how many of them you have observed in your own body.

The rule is that if you check even just one of these 5 indicators, you should consider that your body has an EXCITED nervous system. If you do not check any of the 5 indicators you should consider that your body has a PASSIVE nervous system.

For example, if you only mark *one* of the five indicators on the list (such as being a light sleeper), this would mean that your nervous system is in a state of constant alert to "fight or flee", which is a characteristic of the EXCITED nervous system. Further, if you check two of the indicators (and so on), you would have a greater and greater degree of excitement and be that much more inclined towards having an EXCITED nervous system.

Under no circumstances should you conclude that you have a nervous system that is partly EXCITED and partly PASSIVE. There will always be an inclination either toward PASSIVE or EXCITED and what you ultimately want to discover is which one is more dominant. This test will help discover that. The reality is that we all have both a PASSIVE and an EXCITED side to our nervous system.

THE POWER OF YOUR METABOLISM

But you always find that there is a side that tends to be more active than the other, and that's what you want to know. Remember we are talking about your body and not you. Your body is your body and you are <u>you</u>.

Now, looking at the five indicators in the following table, select how many of these you have observed in your body:

EXCITED NERVOUS SYSTEM INDICATORS	
# 1	**I HAVE TROUBLE DIGESTING RED MEAT (IF YOU DO NOT CONSUME RED MEAT TRY TO IMAGINE WHAT WOULD HAPPEN IF YOU DID)**
# 2	**CONSUMING SATURATED FAT OR FATTY FOODS SUCH AS PORK CHOPS OR FRIED FOODS CAN CAUSE INDIGESTION**
# 3	**IF I EAT LATE AT NIGHT IT UPSETS MY DIGESTION**
# 4	**IF I EAT AFTER CERTAIN HOUR AT NIGHT I WILL HAVE TROUBLE FALLING ASLEEP**
# 5	**I HAVE A "LIGHT SLEEP" AND EXTERNAL NOISES CAN AWAKEN ME EASILY**

What was your score? If you checked one or more of these five indicators you should consider that your body has an EXCITED nervous system. If you did not mark any of the 5 indicators you have a PASSIVE nervous system.

Let us now take a look at what would be the recommend types of foods that you should consume as part of your 2x1 or 3x1 Diet for best results.

These would be the basic, recommend food selections when following your 2x1 or 3x1 Diet based on your nervous system type:

RECOMMENDED FOOD SELECTION	
EXCITED	**PASSIVE**
A DIET WITH AN ABUNDANCE OF VEGETABLES AND SALADS	A CARNIVOROUS DIET
MODERATE CONSUPTION OF "WHITE PROTEINS" WHICH ARE LOW IN FAT SUCH AS CHICKEN, TURKEY AND FISH	RED MEAT, PORK, FATTY FISH SUCH AS SALMON, TUNA AND SARDINES
SMALL PORTIONS OF LOW FAT CHEESES	HIGHER CONSUMPTION OF CHEESES
EGGS: BOILED, SCRAMBLED OR AS AN OMELET BUT NOT FRIED	EGGS: COOKED ANY WAY IS FINE (INCLUDING FRIED)
SALADS AND VEGETABLE JUICES HIGHLY RECOMMENDED	VEGETABLES AND GREENS RECOMMENDEN WITH MEATS OR FISH
LIMIT SALT AND SALTY FOODS	CURB SUGAR INTAKE, SWEET FRUIT, AVOID BREADS OR FLOUR, WHEAT AND CORN
A DIET LOW IN REFINED CARBOHYDRATES	A DIET LOW IN REFINED CARBOHYDRATES

Someone who has an EXCITED nervous system will benefit greatly with the 2x1 or 3x1 Diet by making correct selections of foods that are low in fat and salt.

It is vital that the person who has an EXCITED nervous system chooses the correct type of protein (particularly meat and cheese) and avoids fatty or fried foods or food with a high salt content, since these are foods that stimulate the nervous system. For example, the 2x1 Diet for an EXCITED nervous system would look something like this:

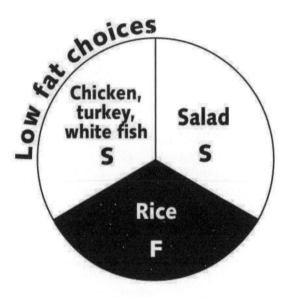

Note that for an EXCITED nervous system it would be best to cook your meat on the grill. If you grill or steam your food, you will be able to prevent excess fat from further stimulating your system. Fried meat, pork or beef (red meat) would not be a good choice for someone with an EXCITED system. However, lean proteins including white meat (such as chicken and turkey) and fresh fish (such as tilapia, cod, or grouper) would be ideal for your body type. . Make it a point not to fry any of the food you eat, as doing so will add quite a bit of extra fat that will negatively affect your system.

Someone with an EXCITED nervous system should also avoid fatty fish like salmon and tuna for the same reason. Certain seafood or shellfish such as shrimp, lobster, clams or oysters are also stimulating to the nervous system and should be reduced to prevent further EXCITMENT and thus, have a more efficient metabolism. Moreover, the EXCITED system tends to retain liquids and suffer from high blood pressure, so be sure to avoid salt and salty foods as well.

Those of us who have a PASSIVE nervous system (like me) on a 2x1 Diet can afford to combine protein that is higher in fat content and have their plate look like this:

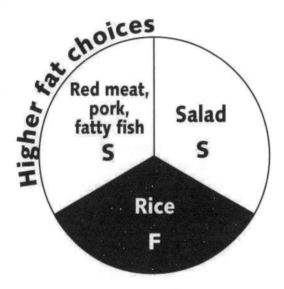

Those who have a PASSIVE nervous system tend to suffer from low blood pressure, as opposed to high blood pressure like an EXCITED nervous system. Salt, in the case of a PASSIVE nervous system, will actually make the body feel better. However, keep in mind that if you have a PASSIVE nervous system but are overweight or obese you may still have high blood pressure due to the fact that excess fat is a major contributing factor to high blood pressure. For this case, you should avoid salt. What really makes a person with a PASSIVE nervous system fat is not the consumption of fat but primarily starches (bread, pizza, cookies, etc.), sugar, sweet fruits, rice and potatoes which will ultimately raise the body's insulin production.

When the nervous system is excited by stimulants (coffee, chocolate, sugar, sweets, nicotine, etc.), it will cause havoc to the body's hormonal system and end up hurting the person's metabolism and health.

While working with thousands of people in my practice who have been helped by the NaturalSlim system, we found that when this data on food choices is correctly applied to the type of nervous system (passive or excited) a particular person has, improvements in the individual's health and energy levels can be impressive. We constantly see cases of people who were once very ill or depressed those "miraculously" improves or no longer have the conditions or diseases they once suffered from, simply by selecting the right foods based on their type of nervous system. This led me to the inevitable conclusion that many health problems and even "metal illnesses" or behavioral problems stem from an improper selection of foods neglecting the needs for that particular type of nervous system.

It is interesting to observe how when an individual correctly applies the 2x1 or 3x1 Diet with their own type of nervous system in mind, their energy will return, their sleep will greatly improve, they will no longer be depressed, and for some, any prescription drugs they were once taking will be deemed no longer necessary by their doctors. And of course, they will slim down!

"ATTENTION DEFECIT AND/OR HYPERACTIVITY"

Unfortunately, many children are quickly diagnosed with modern mental illness like "Attention Deficit" or "hyperactive", the so-called mental diseases are based on opinions and there is no physical test that offers reliable scientific proof (laboratory tests, x-ray, electrocardiogram, etc.) of such a disease. You should also know that the theory of the "chemical brain imbalances" that the promoters of these diseases describe has never been proven. I fear that the children who are victims of these psychiatric diagnoses are often suffering from hereditary EXCITED nervous systems and their parents, due to ignorance, allow them to have a diet that contains stimulants such as sugar, sweets, fat and salt. In many cases these children drink soft drinks (Coca-Cola, Sprite, etc.), which is actually "liquid candy", because one of these drinks can contains up to 39 grams of sugar. It is sad that we have to resort to drugging our children with psychotropic medications such as Ritalin, Adderall, Concerta and others, which are equivalent to street drugs such as cocaine. They could just simply provide the types of food that would effectively calm an EXCITED nervous system, which could handle the problem in a much healthier way.

When the nervous system is too excited the person or the child cannot concentrate their attention because the body is in a state of total uncontrolled nervousness. The EXCITED nervous system is what the body uses in a situation where it should "fight or flight". In other words, it is in control of the body's defense systems for any possible threat that may come up. Note that when the nervous system is overly excited, the body's senses (sight, sound, smell, touch) will sharpen during a state of danger or emergency. If you have children with "attention deficit" or "hyperactive" problems, please review their diet and other factors that may be contributing to an EXCITED nervous system. Some of the other factors that may negatively affect this type of nervous system include the following: *candida albicans* yeast infection (candidiasis), gluten intolerance (the protein found in wheat, bread, pizza, etc.), allergies to dyes or preservatives, heavy metal poisoning, contamination with pesticides, hormonal problems, diet high in sugar or other real medical, nutritional or environmental causes that could be hidden by a diagnosis or label that is, once again, not based on any verifiable scientific evidence.

You can find more information regarding this topic and the possible causes of behavioral problems by visiting Dr. Mary Ann Block's website below:

www.blockcenter.com

You can also learn about your rights as a parent in regard to psychiatric drugs or treatment by visiting the following site:

www.CCHR.org

Anyway, the most important thing is that you observe the results of your decisions about food and about your "lifestyle" to make sure you are making the best decisions for your health and metabolism. All the knowledge in this book is aimed at obtaining positive results. If you see that you have had good results and then notice that your progress has stopped, simply take corrective action and re-do what was previously working. The most important thing in the process of regaining or improving health, energy and metabolism is to observe the results to determine what works best for you.

We are not all the same!

WHAT MIGHT HAPPEN

Now it's time to let you know that when you start applying the information that you've learned about your metabolism and the 2x1 or 3x1 Diet you could start to feel significant changes in your body. The changes that you experience may not be very pleasant at the beginning. If you make the decision to implement this information as a new lifestyle, I guarantee that you will notice a remarkable improvement in your health, diabetes, hypothyroidism and your overall energy.

There is a law of physics that says that for every ACTION there is always a REACTION. This law of physics also applies to the concepts that are talked about in this book. As you start making changes, you could start experiencing reactions that may be unpleasant at first as your body adjusts to the new diet and daily routine.

It's like what happens when an inactive person decides to start exercising. Normally when someone who isn't used to exercising starts being active, they can feel a lot of muscular pain, often to the point that they feel very sore after the first day of exercise. The person did the action (worked out) and produced a reaction (muscular pain).

When you start applying the concepts that are explained in this book, the types of reactions that you could feel in your body are going to depend on the current state of your body. If you are in relatively good shape (hydrated, little yeast, little stress, not ill) you will only experience pleasant reactions such as: more energy, less hunger pains, better quality of sleep, weight loss, and more emotional stability.

However, if you aren't in very good shape (hypothyroidism, diabetes, high blood pressure, dehydrated, excess yeast, and overweight) you could experience one or several unexpected and unpleasant reactions that may worry you if you don't know about them beforehand. This is why I've written this chapter; to warn you about the changes or reactions that you could experience as a result of making changes in your diet and lifestyle with the information in this book.

The good news is that all of the negative reactions (pain, itchiness, redness of skin, drowsiness, and negative changes in laboratory analyses) that you might experience after starting this program ARE TEMPORARY. The reactions eventually disappear. Naturopaths call it a "healing crisis", which means that the human body always worsens briefly before improving.

What might bother you even more is that I don't have the ability to predict and tell you what kinds of things could happen to you in this change process that you are about to start. This chapter was written recently because many people started calling me alarmed about unexpected reactions that they had experienced after changing their diet and applying the concepts that are explained in *The Power of Your Metabolism*. Note that these are things that "could happen". There isn't any way of knowing how you will be affected because we don't know every detail of your body, which naturally isn't the same as anybody else's body.

After having helped more than hundreds of thousands of people slim down with the NaturalSlim system and after having sold over 1 million copies of this book and listened to the feedback, I don't think there are any more situations that we haven't experienced. What I'm sharing with you here is what we've discovered in the last 20 years with respect to the reactions or unexpected changes that you could experience. It is probable that you won't experience anything unpleasant, only improvements. However, I'd like to prepare you so that if you happen to experience an unexpected or unpleasant side effect you won't be surprised.

When you start drinking enough water and changing your eating habits by following the 2x1 or 3x1 Diet you will be affecting and creating changes in your hormonal system. You will also be creating possible reactions if your body is severely infected by the *candida albicans* yeast, as the majority of people who are overweight, diabetic, or have hypothyroidism usually are.

Things that could happen to you but may not happen at all are the following:

HEADACHES, SINUSITIS, MIGRANES, DIARRHEA, EXTREME EXHAUSTION OR ITCHINESS:
Even though it doesn't seem like your body could be severely infected with the *candida albicans* yeast, believe me that it is. Over the years, I've seen thousands of people experience the unpleasant side effects that the *candida* colony causes when it starts to decompose in their bodies. The technical term for all of the unpleasant side effects that can be caused by the decomposing yeast is the "Herxheimer reaction". In the 1920's, a German doctor named Karl Herxheimer described the reactions (headache, inflammation, etc.) that patients with syphilis were suffering from after receiving medication and before completely recovering. In the case of the people who are overweight, diabetic, or suffer from hypothyroidism, toxins that are released from the decomposing yeast usually cause these negative reactions. The most common reactions are headaches, sinusitis, migraines, drowsiness or physical exhaustion, redness of skin and itchiness. The redness of the skin will last a few hours at most. The rest are temporary reactions and go away in just a few days. The number of days that the side effects can last depends on how infected your body is with the *candida* yeast.

RISE IN CHOLESTEROL

If you have laboratory tests done within a few days of having begun the 2x1 or 3x1 Diet, you may find that your cholesterol levels are higher than usual. No need to panic, it is temporary. Sometimes we forget that cholesterol is an essential part of all of the cells in our body including fat cells. When you start making changes to improve your metabolism and you start slimming down quickly, you can lose up to 3 pounds of fat each week. All of the fat that is being broken down <u>contains cholesterol</u> and your cholesterol levels can reflect an increase, but this is due to the fact that the fat cells that are being broken down from weight loss are releasing cholesterol into the blood stream. This temporary increase in cholesterol doesn't have anything to do with the fact that you are eating eggs or meat in the 2x1 or 3x1 Diets. The reality is that the main source of cholesterol that is detected in our blood is the cholesterol that is produced every day in our liver, not the cholesterol that we consume through foods (read the chapter THE TRUTH ABOUT CHOLESTEROL). You can increase your cholesterol levels dramatically if you eat too much of foods like wheat bread; even though it doesn't have cholesterol, your liver can still turn it into cholesterol. Your body produces cholesterol in response to an increase in your glucose levels caused by consuming refined carbohydrates (bread, flour, rice, sugar, etc.). Shortly after starting the recommended diet, you'll notice that your cholesterol will go down to normal levels, but at first it could temporarily increase.

INCREASE IN HEPATIC ENZYMES:

The hepatic (liver) enzymes are substances that show a certain amount of cellular destruction in the liver. Doctors periodically have lab tests done to measure the hepatic enzymes because they reveal the state of the liver. It just so happens that the liver is the favored organ of the *candida albicans* yeast, which infects people who are overweight, diabetic, or have hypothyroidism. This is because the yeast needs the mineral iron in order to reproduce and the liver has more iron than any other organ in the body. This is why anemia (iron deficiency) used to be treated by eating substantial amounts of liver. When you have an infection with the *candida albicans* yeast, it is generally throughout your entire system, but your liver is always the organ that is most affected by this parasite.

Candida albicans is bright white yeast. The word *albicans* comes from the word "albino", which means "white in color". Funeral embalmers have found that when they are working with an obese person their internal organs are always covered with what seems to be a white powder. They have noticed that the organ that is most affected by the white powder (*candida albicans*) is the liver. When an overweight person starts decreasing their intake of refined carbohydrates and starts adding natural foods to their diet that kill yeast, like coconut oil, they may notice that their lab tests show an increase in their hepatic enzymes. This increase usually is temporary and could be caused by the damage to the liver cells that were attacked by the yeast. As the yeast starts to die, its "roots" are destroyed, which causes the cellular enzymes in the liver (where the "roots" of the yeast are embedded) to spread into the bloodstream. This process is what temporarily increases your hepatic enzyme levels.

OTHER SYMPTOMS OR SIDE EFFECTS:
It is impossible to predict everything that you could experience when you are following the 2x1 or 3x1 Diets, especially if you are also starting to use the natural supplements like organic coconut oil that kill yeasts, bacteria, parasites or viruses. We all have different bodies and have different levels of infections of parasitic organisms (yeast, bacteria, parasites, viruses). When you begin making changes to your diet and lifestyle you could feel some unpleasant or unexpected side effects. The majority of people only notice an increase in their energy levels, faster fat loss, and they even start sleeping better. However, throughout the past 20 years, I have seen everything; dizziness, irregular heartbeat, redness of skin back pain, swelling in the legs, phlegm, mucus, vaginal discharge, bloody nose, etc. ALL of these symptoms are temporary, and they go away in a few days. What is important is that you shouldn't be surprised if one or several of them happen to you. There is no need for you to become alarmed or stressed if you experience one of these side

effects. In many ways it is a good sign because you can be assured that you are attacking the yeast. The *candida* is being killed, decomposing, and leaving your body, which is exactly what we want to have happen.

NATURAL AIDS FOR YOUR METABOLISM

Need Help?

The following chapters will cover the importance of various supplements that have been found to greatly improve the function of the metabolism. Should you have any questions about these supplements or where to obtain them, please use the below contact information - our *Certified Metabolism Consultants* are ready to answer your questions!

If you are considering purchasing any of the supplements mentioned here, we recommend that you first complete a Metabolism Evaluation questionnaire. This is a free service to ensure you are getting the correct supplements your body needs in order to effectively improve your metabolism.

To get started, either call or email us using the below information. We look forward to speaking with you!

Phone: 888-574-8438
Email: Info@relaxslim.com
Website: www.us.NaturalSlim.com

DISCOVERIES OF NATURAL SUBSTANCES

Various natural substances have been discovered that help improve or recover the metabolism. They are substances that are extracted from foods, herbs or plants that have a positive effect on your energy and help fight a "slow metabolism".

The scientific discoveries that have been made on some of these natural substances are relatively new. This is the case with the natural substances called "adaptogens[28]", which were originally discovered and researched in Russia.

The others are natural substances that have been known about for hundreds of years like magnesium, zinc or selenium, but there have been recent discoveries as to their importance in improving the metabolism.

The medications that have been developed to help you slim down, are really just chemicals that are looking to block fat or speed up the metabolism, but they do it in a way that isn't very natural for your body. That's why those medications always bring some sort of unpleasant side effects along with them. They are chemicals that don't belong in your body. Recently, the manufacturer of the doctor prescribed, weight loss medication, Xenical, that has been on the market for quite a number of years, got approval from de Food and Drug Administration to sell an over-the-counter (without prescription) version of their Xenical medicine called "Alli". It was a brilliant marketing scheme that will help them make billions of dollars at the expense of those naive consumers that don't know

---

[28] Adaptogen - a natural substance that allows the body to counter adverse physical, chemical or biological stressors by raising resistance toward such stress, thus allowing the organism to "adapt" to the stressful circumstances. Adaptogens are natural herb product that increases the body's resistance to stresses such as trauma, anxiety and bodily fatigue.

THE POWER OF YOUR METABOLISM

about their metabolism. The truth is there are no "miracle pills" out there anywhere. This new over-the-counter medication, Alli, works by blocking all the fats from entering the body and thus the person using it will have a lot of fat coming out of their rear end. But, the problem here is that this substance will block ALL fats indiscriminately and that means that it will also block all the "good fats" that are part of our daily vitamin needs like vitamins A, E and D. That means that you will actually be depriving your body of some essential vitamins while trying to lose weight. Well, that will not work for you.

On the other hand, supplements that are formulated based on natural substances, work in favor of your body and are accepted by your cells, without causing side effects and yet are very effective. That's why I always recommend the use of natural supplements instead of medications.

ADAPTOGENS: THE RUSSIAN SECRET

From 1947 to 1991, there was a period called the Cold War between the United States and Russia. There was an extremely hostile and competitive atmosphere. These two powerful nations were competing at all levels to win alliances in their respective ideologies.

At that time, the Russians tried to show the rest of the world that their technology, military power, physical and sports abilities were the best. Both nations competed in a race of outer space launchings and nuclear technology. In the area of sports and international athletic competitions, the Russians and their allies stood out as outstanding athletes and sportsmen. They especially showed that they had great physical strength and resistance that was unmatched. At the Olympic Games, the Russian athletes always ended up earning many of the top awards.

Part of the Russians athletic success was due to their use of the "adaptogens". The term "adaptogen" was created by the Russians to describe a group of natural substances that have certain special qualities. They are substances that help the human body adapt to conditions of internal and external stress. They are substances that help the body resist situations of stress that would normally have a negative effect on its functioning.

Adaptogens aren't anything like stimulating substances such as caffeine, guarana[29] or ephedrine[30]. Adaptogens are substances that

---

[29] Guarana – A Brazilian berry that contains approximately three times more caffeine than coffee beans. It is used as a stimulant in many sport and weight loss supplements.

[30] Ephedrine - is commonly used as a stimulant or appetite suppressant. It is derived from various plants in the genus Ephedra. The Chinese herb "Ma huang" contains ephedrine.

help the body achieve an ideal balance of internal energies. For example, a natural adaptogen substance tends to lower blood pressure if a person is suffering from high blood pressure. But, this same adaptogen also has the effect of increasing blood pressure if a person has low blood pressure. In other words, the adaptogens "adapt" to the body and contribute to it attaining a more balanced state of cellular function.

There are natural substances that lower blood pressure, like garlic. There are also substances that increase blood pressure, like caffeine or salt. However, adaptogens tend to stabilize blood pressure and the other functions of the body. It is said that adaptogens are "bidirectional" because they work in opposite directions depending on what the need is. This means that they speed up body systems that are very slow (for example, a "slow metabolism"), while slowing and calming down the conditions of emotional stress that obesity has been known to cause.

Adaptogens are natural substances that regulate the internal chemistry of your body in the necessary direction to achieve balance. They increase your body's resistance to stressful situations (being overweight, physical weakness, tiredness, emotional stress, etc.). They give the impression of being "intelligent" substances that cause an increase or decrease of whatever is necessary in your body so as to achieve a better level of adaptation as well as physical, mental and emotional equilibrium.

The Russians conducted secret scientific studies for many years on adaptogens with the idea of gaining an advantage with their soldiers, athletes and astronauts. They did extensive studies with their populations to determine the qualities and effects of adaptogens. The Russian state and only their contracted scientists worked on them and kept these studies secret. The athletes and astronauts secretly used adaptogens to gain more power, better physical strength, mental concentration, coordination and shorter reaction time.

On December 25, 1991, the Soviet Union collapsed as a nation, and the communist party that had been dominating Russia for so many generations lost its control on the Soviet state. That day the Soviet Union dissolved into independent countries and the scientists that had been secretly working with the adaptogens were left without jobs. Many of these scientists emigrated to Europe or the United States, and they took the information that they had learned about the amazing adaptogens with them.

There are more than 3,700 herbs on our planet that have been classified and documented as natural based on their individual properties. However, only 11 of them are considered "adaptogens". In order for a type of herb or plant to be considered an adaptogen, it must have the special characteristic of being able to work in two opposite directions according to what the body needs. In other words, it must have the characteristic of being bidirectional in the way it works. Only 11 of the herbs or plants on the planet fulfill this requirement.

The adaptogens that interest us are the ones that have effects of improving our metabolism and whose qualities contribute to burning fat, controlling stress, reducing inflammation, increasing energy and physical resistance, natural antidepressant effects, and improve our immune system. Some of them include *rhodiola rosea, rhododendron caucasicum, rhaponticum carthamoides* and *ashwagandha.* They are odd names because they are from their botanic origin.

The qualities of these natural adaptogens are very impressive. When you use them along with a 2x1 or 3x1 Diet, in addition to other good habits like drinking a lot of water to improve hydration, you will notice a significant improvement in your metabolism and energy. You'll see results that are reflected in your energy levels and in your clothing, since they will keep fitting looser and looser.

DOCTOR ZAKIR RAMAZANOV

Learning and informing ourselves about these Russian discoveries on adaptogens couldn't have been made possible without the outstanding help and knowledge of Dr. Zakir Ramazanov.

Dr. Ramazanov was one of the main scientists that took part in the secret Russian studies on adaptogens. Through Dr. Ramazanov we have been able to learn about the qualities of these incredible natural substances, adaptogens.

Dr. Zakir Ramazanov was a Russian professor in plant biochemistry and molecular biology. He studied the qualities of different plant extracts, herbs and algae at an in-depth level. Dr. Ramazanov wrote and published hundreds of scientific articles and various books on the topics of adaptogens and algae. Zakir Ramazanov has several approved patents in the field of biotechnology, plant biochemistry, molecular biology and in various active plant compounds. Dr. Ramazanov was a professor at the Technological Institute, University of Spain at Madrid, Louisiana State University and a Chief Scientist at the Russian Academy of Science.

His accomplishments include having been recognized for his work on the subject of growing natural organisms at the MIR Russian Space station.

Dr. Ramazanov is the co-author of various books, including the following:

ARCTIC ROOT "Rhodiola Rosea, The Powerful New Ginseng Alternative" (1998)

"Effective Natural Stress & Weight Management using Rhodiola Rosea and Rhododendron Caucasicum" (1999)

"Rhodiola Rosea for Chronic Stress Disorder" (2002)

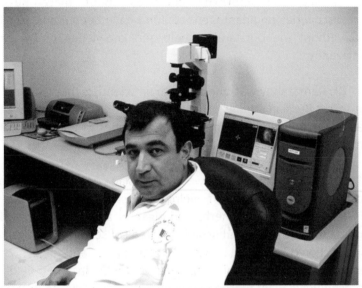

DR. ZAKIR RAMAZANOV

Doctor Ramazanov developed new and ingenious systems for cultivating adaptogen herbs in organic environments with controlled climates. This has allowed for a better yield of the active extracts of these amazing herbs to benefit mankind.

Zakir Ramazanov was one of those few scientists that was totally focused on the discovery and scientific study of natural substances that have the ability to improve our health, energy and emotional state. For me, it was a privilege and an honor to have his expert advice in the areas of using adaptogens to improve the human metabolism. His recommendations about the quality requirements and correct dosage of using the different adaptogens were incredibly valuable. Dr. Zakir's opinions were always backed up by copies of scientific studies that proved the effectiveness of the substances.

The use of adaptogens has brought to the science of the human metabolism a new hope for improving both health and the metabolism.

In late 2006, Dr. Zakir Ramazanov died unexpectedly while in Palma de Mayorca, Spain. For the scientific community, it was an irreparable loss. However, Zakir left behind a legacy of knowledge about the qualities and use of natural substances like the Russian adaptogens and seaweeds. Today, hundreds of thousands of people around the world enjoy the benefits of improved health conditions that these natural substances provide, while traditional medicine only provides medications that simply reduce symptoms.

Zakir was interested in discovering natural substances that helped solve the different causes of sicknesses and conditions. He dedicated his life to the search and discovery of these natural substances that could solve health problems. His scientific research led to the discoveries of natural substances that help solve conditions of being overweight, obesity, depression, hypothyroidism, lack of energy and a slow metabolism.

The last product that Dr. Zakir Ramazanov formulated using adaptogens was the product called RelaxSlim. The success stories from the people that have used this nutritional supplement are really impressive. This product, RELAXSLIM, has all of the accumulated experience and scientific knowledge of Dr. Ramazanov in its formula. The people that use it say that they notice an improvement in their metabolism and in various other conditions like diabetes, thyroid gland problems, and lack of energy, even depression. This product really helps with controlling stress and anxiety. Others find that for the first time, they can slim down without much effort and without the characteristic tiredness that comes along with a "slow metabolism".

Even though Dr. Zakir Ramazanov isn't with us anymore, he left us with the best of his knowledge. His life-long dedication and discoveries in the natural substances field have contributed to our world in such a way that we will benefit forever. His research and scientific successes supporting good health for all humankind truly have an eternal quality.

ADAPTOGEN: RHODIOLA ROSEA

All adaptogens are natural substances with very unique qualities. However, one of the most studied adaptogens, that has also appeared the most in medical news, has been the herb called *rhodiola rosea*. Some years ago, an article came out in *Time* magazine that boasted about how it was "the natural antidepressant of the future."

This plant grows at altitudes between 11,000 to 18,000 feet above sea level. Its yellow flowers smell similar to roses and that's where it gets its name "rosea". It is a type of plant that grows in inhospitable places (where living isn't very easy), and perhaps that is why it developed natural compounds having qualities that increase cellular energy and that make it possible to survive.

Rhodiola is an extraordinary medicinal plant. It was one of the plants considered a "military secret" by the Russians during the Soviet regime. This plant's qualities have been the object of extensive studies.

The adaptogen *rhodiola* has a very old story that includes Chinese emperors ordering special expeditions for what they called the "golden root" or "arctic root". The Chinese considered *rhodiola* a source of well-being and enhanced sexual performance. The use of this plant is documented in the oldest Chinese medical texts, where it was used to fight all types of illnesses.

In 1947, a scientist from the Academy of Russian Sciences named Lasarev reported for the first time that this plant, from the Siberian region, had extracts that helped increase the body's resistance to different environmental stress factors.

The Russian studies on *rhodiola rosea* showed that it had an increased level of therapeutic (curative) activity. Even in high doses the *rhodiola* didn't have toxic or adverse secondary effects. However, it did reveal that it increases the body's resistance to various sicknesses, stressful conditions and to emotional depression.

There are more than 200 varieties of the generic *rhodiola*, but the variety called *rhodiola rosea* is the only one that has special qualities as an adaptogen. The active agents of *rhodiola rosea* were identified as *rosavin, rosin, rosarin* and *salidroside*. Real *rhodiola rosea* contains verifiable potencies of these natural compounds that give it its qualities.

The main effects that interest us about *rhodiola rosea* are its proven qualities to fight obesity and depression. These are qualities that have been proven in various studies that the Russian scientists did on the population.

Various American psychiatrists have started using *rhodiola rosea* to treat their patients with depression. The main advantage that the psychiatrists have seen in using this adaptogen is that *rhodiola rosea* controls depression while also helping the person to avoid gaining weight, like many other anti-depressant medications cause. In fact, the *rhodiola* helped the people slim down while controlling their severe stress conditions.

For example, in a controlled study that took place at the State Hospital of the Republic of Georgia (Russia) with 130 overweight participants, those that used the *rhodiola* lost an average of 20 pounds, while the group that took placebos (trick pills) only lost 7 pounds in the same amount of time.

Rhodiola has the ability of activating the enzyme *lipase*[31], which is an enzyme that the body needs to break up accumulated fat. Even without exercising, taking *rhodiola* extracts increases the eliminating fat by up to 9%. Also, studies show that when you

---

31 Lipase - a water enzyme that breaks up the fat molecules.

combine *rhodiola* with moderate exercise, the amount of fat that you lose increases up to an incredible 72% more. This means that for those people who don't exercise, *rhodiola* can help in slimming down, but for those who do exercise, it can do wonders.

Rhodiola has been shown to increase your strength and resistance during exercise. This is due to the increased levels of a substance called ATP (*adenosine triphosphate*)[32]. ATP is a chemical substance that provides energy for the body and that the cells produce as a result of food metabolism. ATP is a concentrated type of chemical energy. The more ATP that is produced in the cells, the more energy and metabolism your body will have.

Also, studies have been done where *rhodiola* has been shown to have qualities of increasing sexual potency as often in men as in women. In men it was proven that the majority of those who used *rhodiola rosea* significantly lowered their erectile dysfunction and premature ejaculations. These findings support the ancient Russian tradition, from hundreds of years ago, when newlyweds would receive a little jarful of *rhodiola rosea* as a gift to guarantee fertility.

One of the most beneficial effects of *rhodiola rosea* is its ability to lower the *cortisol* hormone levels that the body produces when under stressful conditions. The hormone *cortisol* has the effect of accumulating fat, especially in the areas of the abdomen and hips. This is how we know that stress makes us gain fat. *Rhodiola* has the effect of reducing the body's *cortisol* production and helps even those people who are under severe stress to slim down.

Rhodiola rosea has various other helpful qualities. The most important effects that it has in improving the metabolism have been

---

32 ATP (adenosine triphosphate) - is a substance that the body produces that is most important as a "molecular currency". ATP transports chemical energy within cells for the metabolism. It is a form of chemical energy used by the body.

mentioned. However, the following list of qualities is the complete list:

Anti-arrhythmia (stabilizing heartbeats)
Anti-depressant
Anti-stress
Anti-fatigue
Increases energy
Helps people with Parkinson's
Detoxification of the liver
Improves mental alertness
Improves sexual function
Improves memory
Improves the learning capacity
Improves the ability to concentrate
Burns fat

The use of *rhodiola rosea* also has the effect of improving the quality of your sleep. It is a fact that high levels of *cortisol,* produced during times of stress, prevent people from sleeping properly. People with high levels of *cortisol* in their blood suffer from insomnia and they wake up tired in the morning. *Rhodiola rosea* has the effect of controlling and reducing the production of *cortisol* in the body, and when you use this adaptogen it allows you to start sleeping much better.

The qualities of the adaptogen *rhodiola rosea* have turned it into a valuable aid in the fight against a "slow metabolism" as well as the various other causing factors of a "slow metabolism", like stress.

ADAPTOGEN: RHODODENDRON CAUCASICUM

This next adaptogen was discovered hundreds of years ago in Georgia, which was once part of the Soviet Union. The inhabitants of this region have been drinking *rhododendron caucasicum* tea for many generations. The "alpine tea" that is prepared with *rhododendron caucasicum* is one of their oldest traditions.

According to the most recent statistics, there were more than 23,000 residents over 100 years of age living in Georgia. This represents a high percentage of long-living inhabitants when we consider that the state of Georgia only has 3.2 million residents. The people in this region who are 100 years old or older are almost 1% of the population. Even though tests haven't been done, the general population believes that drinking *rhododendron caucasicum* tea everyday is what allows them to live for so long.

In Russia it was discovered that *rhododendron caucasicum* has qualities that fight asthma attacks and allergies. *Rhododendron caucasicum* blocks the inflammatory action of arachidonic acid, which is a natural compound found in red meats (beef and pork) and some oils. Thus, it has an anti-inflammatory and pain-relieving effect.

We know from scientific studies carried out by the Russians, that *rhododendron caucasicum* has various unique qualities within its class. The proven qualities of this adaptogen are:

Speeds up the elimination of fats in the body
Increases blood flow to the muscles
Increases blood flow to the brain
Increases physical ability and mobility
Helps with mitral valve (heart) conditions
Fights the hardening of the arteries

Fights arteriosclerosis
Detoxification of the body
Protecting effect on blood vessels
Reduces uric acid in Gout[33] conditions
Works as an antidepressant
Inhibits colon cancer
Improves efficiency of the cardiovascular system
Antibacterial qualities
Lowers cholesterol
Lowers blood pressure
Reduces arthritis pain
Reduces or eliminates chest pains
Has an antioxidant effect

Using *rhododendron caucasicum* increases body temperature, stimulates thirst and causes sweating. This effect increases the elimination of toxins in the body and therefore boosts the metabolism. These detoxifying qualities of *rhododendron caucasicum* are what have promoted its popularity as a natural agent in fighting rheumatism arthritis and Gout.

One of its main qualities, the acceleration of the elimination of body fat, is what interests us the most. In one of the studies that the Russian scientists did, it was found that the use of *rhododendron caucasicum* increased the elimination of fat from 15% to 20% when compared to the people in the study that didn't use this adaptogen. This accelerating fat loss effect, makes it so that a person slims down faster than if they hadn't used it.

---

[33] Gout- a medical condition characterized by abnormally elevated levels of uric acid in the blood and recurring attacks of painful joint inflammation (arthritis).

ADAPTOGEN: ASHWAGANDHA

A shwagandha is an adaptogen that doesn't come from Russia, but originally from India.

In controlled clinical studies, this adaptogen has lowered *cortisol* (the stress hormone) levels up to 26%. *Ashwagandha* does this while at the same time lowering the high blood glucose levels that make us fat. *Ashwagandha* helps maintain glucose levels that are lower than what they would normally be. This helps us slim down. It is also a really big help for diabetics. In one study, using *ashwagandha* helped in controlling diabetics' glucose levels much better than the prescribed medications for this condition.

The people that were using *ashwagandha* in these studies also said that they slept better, felt better and experienced less fatigue.

In reference to boosting the metabolism, the main aid that *ashwagandha* offers us is its ability to increase the conversion of the T4 hormone (produced by the thyroid), into the active T3 hormone, which is the hormone that really increases your metabolism. Many people that suffer from hypothyroidism notice a substantial improvement in their energy levels when they use Ashwagandha.

Ashwagandha tends to prevent the stagnation of the metabolism, which happens when a person has been on a diet for several weeks. Since the body is alive, it adapts to the low glucose levels that the diet causes, and this tends to lower the function of the thyroid gland. In improving the conversion of T4 to T3, *ashwagandha* speeds up the metabolism and prevents stagnation.

This adaptogen also has a calming effect on the nervous system. It has been used in India to treat depression and anxiety. It has also been known to have qualities that are valuable in fighting degenerative sicknesses of the brain and nervous system like Alzheimer[34] and Parkinson's[35].

Ashwagandha has antibacterial (kills bacteria), antifungal (kills yeasts), and also anti-tumor qualities (lowers or prevents incidence of tumors). These qualities were proven in different studies that were done in India.

Ashwagandha is referred to as the "ginseng of India" for its energizing qualities. *Ashwagandha* is a natural aid that has been proven effective against a "slow metabolism".

---

[34] Alzheimer's: degenerative sickness of the brain in which a person progressively loses their memory, speech and capacity to think. The causes of this sickness are unknown. It affects more than 5 million people in the United States and more than 30 million people worldwide.
[35] Parkinson's: degenerative condition of the nervous and muscular systems. People with Parkinson's experience shaking, lack of muscular coordination, difficulty eating, muscular stiffness and other symptoms. The causes of this sickness are unknown.

CAUCASIAN BLUEBERRY LEAVES

The *"caucasian blueberry"* plant is a plant with leaves that contain two natural substances (*chlorogenic* and *caffeic acid*), which have shown in clinical studies that they have the following 3 qualities:

1. Reduces intestinal absorption of glucose
2. Reduces the livers production of new glucose
3. Speeds up the use of blood glucose by the cells

The 3 previous qualities are the exact same strategies that help diabetics control their diabetes and obese people slim down. Weight and obesity problems, just like diabetes, are conditions that exist only because of the excess of glucose and insulin. When the absorption and creation of new glucose is reduced, it leads to weight loss and the control of diabetes. If you also speed up the use of the glucose that is building up in your blood, the effect is even more beneficial. The *blueberry leaves* have this stabilizing and regulating effect on the glucose in the blood.

The Russians and Japanese have been drinking *blueberry leaf* tea for many generations; in fact, this tea is called "diabetic tea" in Japan. This traditional homemade remedy has been used for hundreds of years, even though they didn't exactly know how it worked. It is now known that these two natural substances in blueberry leaves mentioned above causes the positive effects.

The extracts from the *blueberry leaves* that they use today are standardized (controlled to a certain potency) with modern chemical processes that guarantee its effectiveness.

Studies show that the use of the *blueberry leaves* extract also reduces "bad" cholesterol levels (LDL) and triglyceride levels (fat in the blood). This is a marginal benefit that adds to the help that these natural extracts provide to people who want to slim down or control their diabetes.

The *blueberry leaf* extracts that have been the object of studies are known as *caucasian blueberry leaves* and are only grown in Russia. No other variety of common blueberry leaves has been shown to have the necessary potency to achieve these desired effects.

For diabetics and all of those people who want to slim down, the *Caucasian blueberry leaf* extract is a valuable aid.

THE "GUGGUL" SUPPLEMENT

One of the main reasons that people fail in diets is due to the body's capacity to adapt to any change in their food or environment. The human body is an organism that self-regulates by using the hormonal system as a controlling agent.

Glucose is the primary food for all of the cells in your body. When a person starts a diet, the first thing that the body feels is the lower level of glucose. The body's first response to the decrease of glucose is to start breaking its accumulated fat to turn it into glucose to feed the cells. This is part of the body's ability to adapt.

Now, when a diet continues for several weeks, the body notices that the glucose levels continue to be lower than usual. This is a situation that the body seems to interpret as a "time of shortage". Its reaction to the "shortage" is to conserve energy. Apparently, the body does this to improve its possibilities of surviving during a real or supposed food "shortage".

The way that the body conserves energy is by reducing the production of the thyroid hormones to slow down the metabolism. In other words, it reduces the production of the T4 hormone and its product, T3. This slows down the metabolism and conserves energy.

It is inevitable for the body to react in this way when doing any diet system: it lowers the production of the thyroid and along with it the metabolism. It is an automatic mechanism that is designed to survive any shortage situation. Any diet tends to bring along with it a certain reduction of the metabolism.

There are different techniques that are used to prevent the body from slowing the metabolism down during diets. All of these help: drinking a lot of water, exercising, using organic coconut oil and taking powerful vitamins.

Other than these techniques, you can help your body avoid the reduction of the metabolism during a diet by using a natural supplement called *guggul*. This supplement is a resin produced by a tree in India that is known as *"commiphora mukul"* or *"guggulipid"*. Hundreds of years ago, guggul was used in India to fight obesity. They didn't know why it helped fight obesity; all they knew was that it worked.

It was recently discovered that *guggul* stimulates the production of the thyroid gland hormones. This helps increase the production of the T4 and T3 hormones, which prevents the metabolism from slowing down during a diet.

Guggul contains new active substances called *"guggulsterones"*, which reduce "bad" cholesterol levels (LDL), while increasing the proportion of "good" cholesterol (HDL). It is already known that hypothyroidism conditions cause increases in cholesterol. When *guggul* improves the function of the thyroid, it decreases the cholesterol for the same reason. *Guggul* also decreases triglycerides (fat in the blood).

In 1986 the government of India gave manufacturers of natural supplements permission to advertise their products manufactured using *guggul* and to promote them as natural medicines to lower cholesterol.

It is obvious that the benefits that *guggul* provide in reference to slimming down are related to its ability to stimulate the thyroid.

A way to help fight a "slow metabolism" that has been slowed down due to a diet is to take a supplement that contains *guggul*.

ORGANIC COCONUT OIL

Thirty years ago, the news media and medical authorities started a massive campaign to inform the public about the damage that coconut oil could cause. It was then publicized that coconut oil was a saturated fat. They even went as far to say that it raises cholesterol. They said that the public should avoid the consumption of coconut oil at all costs. The campaign was successful and coconut oil disappeared from our diet. Manufacturers that used it in making their products substituted it for soy or corn oil, which was supposedly much better for our health.

At that time there was a coordinated effort and campaign of public relations for soy oil manufacturers to monopolize the oil market. At that time a hysterical media (newspapers, radio, TV) had a field day criticizing the supposed evils of coconut oil. Well, they convinced us that coconut oil was "bad" and that soy oil was "good".

Nowadays, it is known that all of this was a lie, or a serious misunderstanding of the subject. The information that the "experts" told us at that time was wrong.

Coconut oil is a saturated fat. That is true. Now, all saturated fats are not "bad" in the same way that there is "good" and "bad" cholesterol. In the past we thought that all cholesterol was "bad", up until it was discovered that there are significant differences between the two types of cholesterol.

The saturated fat that coconut oil contains is a fat called *medium chain triglycerides*, or MCT's. In fact, it is a type of saturated fat whose molecule is very small and which the body does not use to build more fat. The saturated fat molecules in coconut oil are so small that the body sends them DIRECTLY to the cells to be turned into energy without first going through the liver's filter, which is what happens with all other fats and oils that we eat. Coconut oil contains saturated fats that almost instantly turn into ENERGY. That helps us boost our metabolism and slim down.

Coconut oil has ended up being one of the most valuable substances that there is to help people increase their metabolism and slim down. Notice that weight problems and obesity practically don't even exist in areas like the islands in the Pacific Ocean, where they use coconut oil every day to cook and fry.

For people with hypothyroidism, using coconut oil has been a blessing. This oil increases body temperature to the point where you can actually take your body's temperature and notice the difference. People with hypothyroidism have lower body temperatures because it is a result of a "slow metabolism". The slower your metabolism is, the colder your body will be.

I spent years searching for a natural supplement that would really make a difference to be able to help people with hypothyroidism. I've never seen anything work as effectively to warm the body and boost the metabolism as coconut oil. Even people with hypothyroidism can slim down when they take a dose of coconut oil every day.

CAUTIONS

The coconut oil that you use must be "organic". "Organic" means that the product is certified by an accredited institution that inspects the areas where the product is farmed and processed to guarantee that they have never used pesticides, chemical solvents, preservatives or dyes in the processing or packaging of the crop. When something is "organic", it guarantees its purity.

Coconut oil has a compound called *caprylic acid*. This compound, which is a natural part of coconut oil, has qualities that are of interest to us. The qualities are:

- It is a fungicide and kills yeast like *candida*
- It destroys certain viruses like herpes
- It kills disease causing bacteria
- It detoxifies and helps the body get rid toxins

These qualities help us clean our body of parasitic organisms that cause infections and decrease our metabolism. This is a very good thing. However, the problem lies in that some people are so infected from these organisms that when they use coconut oil they can suffer some severe reactions from the sudden death of the parasitic organisms in their bodies. They are reactions that can be very unpleasant like:

- Headaches
- Diarrhea
- Muscular pain
- Itchy skin
- Mucus in nasal passages

These reactions are caused by the death of the parasitic organisms that live in the body, like the *candida albicans* yeast, bacteria, viruses and parasites that live in the intestines and other organs in the body. The problem is that these parasitic organisms die INSIDE the body. Dying inside of the body causes them to decompose and turn into toxins that cause the body to have unpleasant reactions.

If you start using coconut oil in your diet to boost your metabolism, you might not feel any of these unpleasant side effects. However, you can feel them if your body is heavily infected by any of these organisms. Many, if not all, overweight or obese people are infected with these parasitic organisms like *candida albicans*.

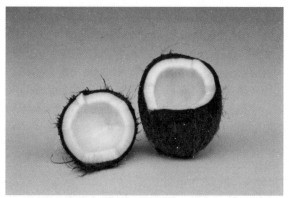

COCONUT IS A NATURAL SOURCE OF MEDIUM CHAIN TRIGLICERIDES
THAT BOOST THE METABOLISM

Coconut oil really works wonders for slimming down. It is something that actually works! However, you do have to know how to use it sensibly and intelligently.

The solution is to start with a low daily dose to give your body the opportunity to get rid of the toxins that have built up from the internal organisms dying. People that have severe *candida albicans* infections (see the section: *CANDIDA ALBICANS*, "THE SILENT EPIDEMIC") should be especially careful not to increase the dosage too quickly.

The key is to GRADUALLY increase your coconut oil dosage. For example, increase your dose by only ½ tablespoon a day each week.

There is a type of coconut oil that is classified as "virgin" that is also "organic". However, when you are using it to speed up your metabolism, it is better to use organic coconut oil as opposed to "virgin" because it doesn't have any flavor and doesn't change the taste of the shakes or other foods that you mix it with. Organic coconut oil has no taste whatsoever.

There are various books written about the qualities of organic coconut oil. In my opinion, the best one is called, *The Coconut Oil Miracle*, written by the naturist Doctor Bruce Fife.

FINAL SUMMARY

No one, not even I, possess 100% of the truth. That's why no one can really claim that their point of view and their opinions are the only correct ones.

I've spent a good part of my life searching for the main factors that cause the condition of a "slow metabolism", which each day produces more and more people with conditions of weight problems or obesity. They are the same factors that to, my understanding; keep many people sick and taking medications.

Even if you don't practice everything that is recommended in this book, it is certain that if you practice the most basic concepts that have been expressed here, you will have positive results. Advice like drinking a lot of water, following a diet low in refined carbohydrates and sugar, taking powerful vitamins and looking for supplements or ways to control your stress levels, will all help you improve your energy levels, metabolism and health.

There are special natural supplements formulated to boost your metabolism like RELAXSLIM, METABOLIC PROTEIN , COCO-10 PLUS and STRESS DEFENDER ANGEL (for natural stress control). However, you don't have to use them to be successful in slimming down and recovering your metabolism. The use of supplements is to make the process easier. Even without using these special supplements, you will notice a significant improvement in your energy levels and your metabolism if you start to apply the recommendations that I have made in this book. I have seen it work for more than hundreds of thousands of people that we have helped with the NaturalSlim system.

If you are curious to know how affected your metabolism is, visit the NaturalSlim System website at www.us.NaturalSlim.com and do the free metabolism test on the main page. This metabolism test was designed with the help of various universities and metabolism specialists. When you finish answering the questionnaire part of the free metabolism test, your percentage of available metabolism should always be 100%, but most likely it won't be a 100%. If your result is, for example, 80%, this means that you have lost the equivalent of 20% of your metabolism. That of course would indicate you have a "slow metabolism".

If you have already failed in many diets and previous attempts, it is possible that you need the help that is provided by the special natural supplements that contain the Russian adaptogens and other substances like CoQ10, L-Tyrosine and others described in this book.

The special supplements like RELAXSLIM, METABOLIC PROTEIN, COCO-10 PLUS and STRESS DEFENDER ANGEL have been created taking into account the main factors that cause a "slow metabolism". These factors include controlling stress, helping the thyroid gland, controlling the *candida albicans* yeast and using adaptogens and special natural substances to increase the metabolism without affecting the nervous system.

Whatever happens, now that you have read this book, you won't be able "unlearn" what you have learned about your metabolism. The knowledge that you now have about the causes of the "slow metabolism" and its solutions compels you to take the responsibility of doing something to better it. People that have a "slow metabolism", due to their lack of knowledge, are victims of their own ignorance about the subject. But, once they know about the causes and solutions to the problem, the only thing that matters is their level of RESPONSIBILITY and their firm decision to do something about it.

Problems don't solve themselves. The problem of a "slow metabolism" is not an exception to this rule. There aren't any "miracles" or "miracle pills". There is only the knowledge and the will to succeed.

If you suffer from diabetes, you have to realize that your life is at stake. Diabetics suffer from more fatal sicknesses than any other part of the population. Most diabetics suffer from high blood pressure, high triglycerides, heart problems, liver problems, diabetic neuropathy, (loss of sensation in nerves), even blindness. Diabetic men many times become sexually impotent. If you want to take control of your diabetes before your diabetes takes away your enjoyment of life, you have to control your intake of refined carbohydrates and sugar. The other recommendations like hydrating your body, taking potent vitamins and using organic coconut oil, all will improve your metabolism and health.

Within the subject of the metabolism, the most important thing is CONSISTENCY. It's having a defined course of action with a strategy that makes sense. For example, I guarantee that if your strategy is to reduce your intake of refined carbohydrates in order to lower your blood glucose levels, you will slim down to where you want to be. Whether you do it quickly or slowly, it's more a question of how many factors you incorporate to boost your metabolism and how many you ignore.

You really don't need an excessive amount of discipline. What you need to have is the right KNOWLEDGE about the situation. If you understand the message that I am trying to give you, you can apply what you have learned and never go hungry. Therefore, you won't have to depend just on discipline.

Don't put too much pressure on yourself, either. You don't need to add any additional stress to your life. Remember that stress makes you fatter! Here, the key to success is to MAKE THE DECISION and then, against all odds, make it happen by applying what you have learned.

Also, if you use the 90/10 rule, you will be successful. The 90/10 rule is the rule of doing things right at least 90% of the time and leaving 10% for the times when you want to be "bad" and eat everything that you desire. If you are overweight or obese, it is only

THE POWER OF YOUR METABOLISM

due to the 50% to 80% of the times that you are doing things incorrectly. Switching to doing things right 90% of the time is a tremendous improvement and doesn't require you to make that big of a sacrifice. We don't want stress we want positive results.

The Power of Your Metabolism is still in your body. Applying what you have learned will help you recover your metabolism to the maximum that is possible for your age. Your metabolism can be improved if you start to cooperate with your body with a new and improved "lifestyle". You still have the potential to improve your metabolism and health. Everyone can improve if they apply this knowledge.

SPECIAL SUPPLEMENTS: THE NATURALSLIM SYSTEM

THE SEARCH FOR WHAT PRODUCES
GOOD RESULTS

These last 20 years of work and the experience of having helped more than hundreds of thousands of people lose weight on the NaturalSlim system have made me learn which techniques work. In the case of NaturalSlim, it was a situation where we either produced positive results in our members, or we would have simply failed as a company. It's true that "happy clients are the best advertising". But it's also true that if what we do in NaturalSlim doesn't produce the expected results, our failure as a company wouldn't take long. The news about the things that don't work, the hoaxes, as well as any hearsay, always spreads faster than any good advertising.

Therefore, I dedicated all those years to observing and isolating those factors that really showed improvement to the metabolism and helped in slimming down. We tried everything! Many times, we found that even though they were techniques that seemed to be very logical, they simply didn't produce results with our members. For a long time, our NaturalSlim system members were parts of a large scale "experiment", where we were interested to find out if a certain natural supplement or nutritional technique that we had researched really worked or not.

We tested hundreds of different natural supplements with NaturalSlim members to determine which ones would produce results and which ones would not. Having the advantage of measuring and weighing the fat levels of hundreds of people each week, we could see if our recommendations of supplements or foods were working or not. As soon as we discovered that a new supplement didn't make a noticeable difference in weekly fat loss, we eliminated it as a possible alternative. Results were the most important thing to our members, and us and finding them included a long process of trial and error and experimentation.

After several years, we successfully identified those natural supplements and diet recommendations that really produced a metabolism increase and consistent fat loss. These days we don't experiment with anything in the NaturalSlim system. We don't need to anymore, because we get uniform results that are good for the majority of our participating members. They say, "if it works, don't change it", and that's why we are now running NaturalSlim only with what has shown to produce good results.

We always keep ourselves up to date on the new discoveries related to the metabolism, but now we aren't in a frantic search for what works and what doesn't work like we were in the beginning. We simply know what works and that when applied you achieve good results.

In addition, we know that there are hundreds of thousands, if not millions of people that need help but are unaware of the causes of "slow metabolism", weight problems and obesity. Some people don't need an intensive and personalized treatment like the one that NaturalSlim offers. Other people live too far from a NaturalSlim office to receive assistance. And there are people who don't have the economic means to pay for an intensive and personalized system like NaturalSlim.

NaturalSlim specializes in "difficult cases" of people that have already "tried everything". We have been successful in this area because generally people that haven't slimmed down in any other system slim down with the NaturalSlim system. It's not that we are doing anything special; it's that we are TEACHING people to apply what will help them recover their metabolism. NaturalSlim has an educational focus where the main aid is the KNOWLEDGE that the person gains to slim down and not go back to gaining weight again. From there the slogan was born: "The weight lost, that stays lost!"

As part of the experience and knowledge gained in NaturalSlim, we learned that the metabolism is lowered due to a variety of factors. There are more than 13 different factors; however, there are four of them that are very important amongst the people that have "slow metabolism". These 4 main factors are:

1. The negative **effect that stress has** and the excessive production of the hormone *cortisol* that causes the buildup of fat and that lowers the metabolism. In other words, stress makes us fat.

2. **Problems with the thyroid gland** and the conversion of the T4 hormone into the active hormone T3. People with hypothyroidism are direct victims of this factor, but it is also a factor for all those people that go on a diet for more than 3 or 4 weeks.

3. **Infections with the *candida albicans* yeast**, whose toxins produce a "slow metabolism", along with a number of symptoms and sicknesses like itchy skin, sinusitis, and migraines.

4. The **wrong diet**, which is too rich in refined carbohydrates (bread, flour, potatoes, sweets, etc.) without adequate hydration (water).

With the idea of offering help to these hundreds of thousands or millions of people that don't need intensive help or that for one reason or another can't go to any of the NaturalSlim centers, we offer our supplements and our metabolism improving system to everybody with Certified Metabolism Consultants over the phone and mailing the system's supplements to your doorstep. One of our slogans is "Eat what you want, lose what you want". This slogan is a true statement because the 2x1 diet that we recommend allows you to eat everything you want. You only have to learn to balance the proportion of the "S" (slimming foods) versus the "F" (fattening foods).

We can improve the three main metabolism-reducing factors (stress, thyroid gland, and *candida albicans*) with two natural supplements called RELAXSLIM and COCO-10 PLUS. We then can improve on the factor of the wrong diet with a whey protein shake called METABOLIC PROTEIN, which is recommended as a breakfast, along with the 2x1 or 3x1 Diet (See the topic: A DIET YOU CAN LIVE WITH).

Stress control can be enhanced with a supplement called STRESS DEFENDER that actually helps you control the negative hormonal effects produced by stressful situations.

With this approach, we do our best to handle the most important obstacles that the body has in order to overcome a "slow metabolism" and slim down while at the same time recovering your metabolism.

I've been researching the components and natural substances of these supplements from the NaturalSlim System for more than 3 years. The consultants of the NaturalSlim system were secretly participating in testing the results and effects that the new substances, like Russian adaptogens, would produce in their bodies. We wanted to offer something that would produce positive results, and the only way to do this was to test the substances on ourselves.

When we discovered the Russian adaptogens, we had the assistance of the late Dr. Zakir Ramazanov, who helped us understand the multiple benefits these substances have for the metabolism and stress control. Dr. Ramazanov helped us find the purest sources, as well as laboratory tested and certified adaptogens (*rhodiola rosea, rhododendron caucasicum, rhaponticum carthamoides "leuza"*). Within the market of supplements and natural ingredients there are some imitations and adulterated substances. The problem is that worldwide, the business ethics aren't much to speak of. Therefore, you have to know the quality of the natural substance, ingredient, or herb that you buy, and make sure that it is certified by specialized laboratories that test its potency and be assured that it is free of pesticides and adulterating toxins.

The point is that there are real solutions to the problem of a "slow metabolism", being overweight or obese. None of these solutions reside in a "miracle pill". The only true solutions have to take into consideration ALL THE FACTORS that either help or reduce the metabolism. We have been experiencing huge successes since this book and these products first came out. It's a joy to see people losing weight and recovering both their metabolism and their health on a daily basis.

Anybody can do it, but it is the KNOWLEDGE that really empowers us to achieve our goals.

THE RELAXSLIM® SUPPLEMENT

We created a supplement, RelaxSlim®, which contains a combination of 21 different natural compounds that have been seen to improve the metabolism. They are natural substances that lower the effects of stress, the growth of the *candida albicans* yeast and provide support for the thyroid gland, which is vital in boosting the metabolism.

This supplement comes in capsules; you take two (2) with your breakfast and two (2) at lunch. Through our search, we found natural substances that contain higher potencies of their active compounds to avoid what would be taking dozens of pills every day that have lower potency.

This supplement contains Russian adaptogens that provide energy, burn fat, and lower the production of the hormone *cortisol*, which is produced by stress and makes us fat. It also contains the vitamins and minerals that prevent the *candida albicans* yeast from reproducing and spreading uncontrollably inside your body. There are also natural supplements like *biotin*, which is part of the B complex vitamins. This vitamin stops the reproductive system of the *candida* yeast and controls its growth.

We also use a relatively high dosage of *niacin* (vitamin B3*)*. Niacin is a fungicide vitamin, or a yeast killer. Niacin also has an antidepressant effect, lowers cholesterol, gets rid of toxins in the body, and breaks up fats. None of this is true with the *niacinamide* that most vitamin manufacturers use. Commercial vitamin manufacturers substitute *niacinamide* (the industry's creation), for *niacin (*vitamin B3**,** a vitamin in its natural state), to prevent *niacin* from causing an unpleasant reaction when reacting with the body's toxins or yeasts. *Niacin* is a detoxifier vitamin. That's why people whose bodies are full of toxins can experience a "niacin flush" in their skin. For example, when there was a nuclear accident in

Chernobyl, Russia in 1986, the people were given a dose of *niacin* (vitamin B3*)* to help extract the radiation that had built up in their bodies. If you start using RelaxSlim® and notice that at times your face turns a reddish color, be assured that you aren't in any danger. Your body is just cleansing itself from the built-up toxins and, with some time, you will stop having these reactions.

RelaxSlim® contains herbs like guggul and the adaptogen ashwagandha, which help the thyroid gland function better. It also contains all of the vitamins and minerals that are essential to the body and to the thyroid, to turn the T4 hormone, that the thyroid produces, into the T3 hormone, that really boosts the metabolism. It contains a natural compound called *"myricetin"*, which in controlled studies has proven to increase the thyroid's absorption of the mineral iodine. It also contains blueberry leaf extracts, which lowers blood glucose levels, which helps you slim down and control diabetes.

The RelaxSlim® supplement has another benefit in the fact that it contains the adaptogen *rhodiola rosea*, which has an anti-stressing, anti-depressing and fat burning effect on the body. This adaptogen, *rhodiola rosea*, also has the effect of increasing your sexual prowess and appetite, as much in men as in women, which is why it has been used in Russia as an aphrodisiac [36] for many generations. There is a tradition in Russia of giving the gift of a little jar of *rhodiola rosea* to newlyweds to guarantee the couple's fertility.

RelaxSlim® also contains adaptogen herbs like *rhaponticum carthamoides (leuza)* and *rhododendron caucasicum*, which increase cellular energy throughout the entire body and also improve intellectual and learning capacity.

---

36 Aphrodisiac - An aphrodisiac is a substance which is used to increase sexual desire. The name comes from the Greek goddess of Sensuality, *Aphrodite*.

In conclusion, RelaxSlim® is the product of 3 years of intense research, tests and consultations with researchers and scientists who know the subject of the metabolism. It doesn't contain any stimulating substances because as we've already seen, stimulating agents, even if they are natural, aren't beneficial in the long run. In fact, they can cause you to feel too stimulated and in a state of nervousness comparable to having drank a few too many cups of coffee. Therefore, we use the anti-depressing, energizing and calming qualities that the adaptogens contain. This is how we boost the metabolism, by cooperating with the body's well-being and energy, and without forcing it.

Bear in mind that although the regular dosage of the RelaxSlim® supplement is two (2) capsules with your breakfast and two (2) at lunch, this doesn't necessarily apply in 100% of cases. We are all a little bit different. The majority, or about 90% of the people, will do well with this dosage but all of us do not have identical bodies or similar metabolisms. Some people will find that the regular dosage of two (2) capsules at breakfast and two (2) capsules at lunch might be too strong for them. When this happens, instead of feeling energized by this supplement you will feel weakened and sleepy. What it means is that the cell's energy is overflowing and that weakens the body. The solution if you feel sleepy or weaken when taking a dosage of two (2) and two (2) is to lower the dosage to one (1) and one (1). When you hit on the right dosage for your body you will feel energized but relaxed.

The contrary is also true in some cases like my own. I could use the regular two (2) capsules and two (2) capsules dosage but my own metabolism is so slow that I do better on three (3) capsules for breakfast and three (3) capsules for lunch. With this higher dosage I feel better, tireless and lose weight easier.

Anyway, you will feel the difference when you do use the supplement RelaxSlim®. Combined with the right diet, like the 2x1 Diet, it really works.

COCO-10 PLUS™

A few years ago, we introduced organic coconut oil to our NaturalSlim system members. It was, without a doubt, one of the most important discoveries in the last 20 years of our history as a weight loss system.

The results were spectacular. People with hypothyroidism, that were losing weight at a slower weekly rate due to their condition, started losing weight at almost double the speed, as soon as they started using organic coconut oil on a daily basis. All of the members that started using organic coconut oil increased their rate of fat loss at their weekly weigh-ins.

From then on, organic coconut oil turned into one of the standard supplements of the NaturalSlim system.

Naturally, if organic coconut oil isn't accompanied with the right diet, it won't give you these results. There are no "miracles". Still, we were seeing if there was a way to improve even further on the organic coconut oil qualities that had already proven to be of benefit.

We saw hundreds of possibilities, but finally we discovered that the supplement CoQ10, which has many clinical studies that prove its ability to boost cellular energy and improve the metabolism, could be what we needed to create a "super organic coconut oil". That's why we did tests, consulted with chemists of natural products, read the studies, and finally created COCO-10 PLUS™.

COCO-10 PLUS™ is a "super coconut oil", because it is a blend of high quality organic coconut oil with the energizing supplement CoQ10 that increases and improves respiratory processes and the oxygenation of your cells. CoQ10 increases the production of the

THE POWER OF YOUR METABOLISM

cellular energy molecule ATP (*"adenosine triphosphate"*). This increases your metabolism.

The Japanese control the production of the CoQ10 supplement worldwide. The Japanese are the ones who discovered the natural fermentation processes that allow this compound to be produced in such huge quantities. It is an expensive supplement!

The CoQ10 supplement is expensive because its worldwide production hardly covers the international demand and that makes it more expensive. In Japan, Germany, Switzerland, Australia and other countries, CoQ10 is used as medical treatment for heart problems.

It turns out that CoQ10 has never been combined with organic coconut oil before. This is why it was a great success since there were dozens of tests done with different brands of CoQ10 to be able to obtain a CoQ10 that would dissolve perfectly inside the organic coconut oil. The purity of the CoQ10 had to be 99% or more to be able to perfectly dissolve in the organic coconut oil. Finally, we did it.

Organic coconut oil has a quality that luckily goes perfectly with CoQ10. Organic coconut oil increases the absorption of the other oils that are combined with it to double the absorption from what is normal. In other words, the organic coconut oil is made up of *medium chain triglycerides (*MCT'S*)* that are sent directly to the cells, without passing through the liver. This makes it so that nothing is wasted or lost between the intake of the coconut oil and what gets to the cells. That's why organic coconut oil goes directly to the cells and its energizing effect isn't delayed.

The pharmaceutical industry is the biggest consumer of organic coconut oil worldwide. They discovered that organic coconut oil is a "carrier oil" that transports everything that is mixed with it inside the cells. That's why pharmaceutical companies purchase thousands of barrels of organic coconut oil; they use it to mix with their medications, that are soluble in oil, to improve absorption and the cellular penetration of their medicines.

This "carrier oil" quality that organic coconut oil has, increases the potency of the dose that we use of CoQ10 in the COCO-10 PLUS™ because as the absorption potential increases to double, the dose of CoQ10 also amounts to double. The CoQ10 combined with the organic coconut oil is really a potent stimulator for the metabolism.

One of the most noticeable effects after using the COCO-10 PLUS™ supplement is the mental clarity that it produces. COCO-10 PLUS™ creates this benefit because in increasing the energy that your cells produce, it also improves the energy production of the brain cells.

You should know that the organic coconut oil that COCO-10 PLUS™ contains changes from liquid to solid form depending on the room temperature. The COCO-10 PLUS™ supplement doesn't need refrigeration because organic coconut oil is very stable and doesn't go bad in a warm environment. If you live in a place where the temperature is colder than 76° Fahrenheit, your COCO-10 PLUS™ will be solid, since the cold solidifies the coconut oil. This doesn't mean that the product is damaged. You just have to warm it up a bit and it will turn into liquid again, so you can mix it in your shake or take it directly in spoonful. If it solidifies because of cold weather put the closed jar under running hot water for a short time and it will become liquid again.

COCO-10 PLUS™ is an important aid especially for people who suffer from hypothyroidism or people who are excessively obese because it boosts the metabolism.

The dose of COCO-10 PLUS™ should be increased gradually. So, the dosages would look something like this:

First week:
MONDAY - ½ tablespoonful
TUESDAY- ½ tablespoonful
WEDNESDAY - ½ tablespoonful
THURSDAY - ½ tablespoonful
FRIDAY - ½ tablespoonful
SATURDAY - ½ tablespoonful
SUNDAY - ½ tablespoonful

Second week:
MONDAY - 1 tablespoonful
TUESDAY - 1 tablespoonful
WEDNESDAY - 1 tablespoonful
THURSDAY - 1 tablespoonful
FRIDAY - 1 tablespoonful
SATURDAY - 1 tablespoonful
SUNDAY - 1 tablespoonful

Third week:
MONDAY – 1½ tablespoonful
TUESDAY - 1½ tablespoonful
WEDNESDAY - 1½ tablespoonful
THURSDAY - 1½ tablespoonful
FRIDAY - 1½ tablespoonful
SATURDAY - 1½ tablespoonful
SUNDAY - 1½ tablespoonful

From 1½ tablespoon a day you would increase the dose to 2 tablespoons a day and so on, increasing by ½ tablespoon each week. You can keep on increasing the dose up to 4 tablespoons a day, when your body allows it. If you start having constant diarrhea, then you have gone over the appropriate dosage for your body and you should reduce your intake of it.

The majority of people do well with 2 tablespoons a day. Remember that we are talking about tablespoonfuls, not teaspoonfuls.

COCO-10 PLUS™ also helps reduce the *candida albicans* yeasts in your body and this boosts your metabolism, which helps you slim down. However, it's very important that you increase your dose of COCO-10 PLUS™ gradually to give your body the opportunity to eliminate the toxins that are produced as a result of killing the yeasts in your body.

METABOLIC PROTEIN™

Nutrition, in general, is a really important factor to boost your metabolism. For people who suffer from a "slow metabolism", breakfast is the most important meal of the day. That is also true for those that are interested in maintaining their weight.

The best way that we have seen to start the day and give your metabolism the impulse to "wake up", is to drink a whey protein shake for breakfast. This doesn't mean that you have to drink a shake every day. You can occasionally have a 2x1 or 3x1 type breakfast with fried or scrambled eggs or an omelet with a little piece of bread. However, a couple of fried eggs could never boost your metabolism like a whey protein shake such as METABOLIC PROTEIN™ would.

METABOLIC PROTEIN™ shakes aren't common shakes like the ones that are sold in natural food stores or the ones that bodybuilders use to increase muscle. They are shakes that are formulated to boost the metabolism. The necessities of a person with a slow metabolism aren't the same as bodybuilders or people who don't have this problem.

METABOLIC PROTEIN™ is a product of advanced nutritional technology. It's what is called a "meal replacement" because it contains ALL of the vitamins and minerals; therefore, the FDA (Food and Drug Administration) requires it to be called a "meal replacement". Common protein shakes aren't "meal replacements" because they aren't complete foods and don't qualify for this classification by the FDA. A common protein shake is a protein "supplement" to supplement a normal diet, but you can't drink it as if it were a complete meal. METABOLIC PROTEIN™ is a "meal replacement". In other words, it is a complete meal. METABOLIC PROTEIN™ can be used to replace dinner if you don't want to eat some other type of food for dinner. Generally, you only drink it once a day for breakfast, but you could repeat its use if necessary. It's a complete meal.

If some days, you decide to have a METABOLIC PROTEIN™ shake in the evening, make sure you don't add a dose of the COCO-10 PLUS™. COCO-10 PLUS™ causes a quick boost to your metabolism and provides energy. You wouldn't want this energy when it is time to go to sleep, because it will wake you up. That's why COCO-10 PLUS™ should be used in the morning or early in the afternoon, but never at night.

Most of the whey shakes that are on the market have another problem, along with not being "meal replacements": they taste bad. This is a real problem because how could you drink a whey protein shake every morning if it turns into a nightmare just to swallow it?

METABOLIC PROTEIN™ tastes good. After hundreds of tests and having tested all of the shakes that are on the market, we can say that you won't find a better tasting shake than METABOLIC PROTEIN™. In fact, it is sold with a "satisfaction guarantee" offer that allows to you return it for complete credit if for some reason you don't like the way it tastes. It comes in three flavors: vanilla, chocolate, and strawberry. Each flavor has its fans. Some people like to add a different touch to the vanilla shake by adding almond extract or cinnamon to it. Everyone is boss when it comes to the subject of flavors. The flavors are a question of personal taste. In tests that we've done, METABOLIC PROTEIN™ had an acceptance rate of more than 95%.

METABOLIC PROTEIN™ contains powerful enzymes [37] that increase the absorption of the whey protein amino acids to up to about 98%. A dose of METABOLIC PROTEIN™ provides a metabolism

---

[37] Enzymes: substances that allow foods to digest more efficiently. It has been discovered that no more than 70 % of the proteins are absorbed, which means that at least 30% is wasted and isn't used by the body.

increase for many hours. The metabolism increase is due to the fact that the amino acids are made entirely (98%) available to the cells as sources of energy. Only 70% or less of common proteins are absorbed when they aren't taken with special enzymes that increase their absorption.

The METABOLIC PROTEIN™ shakes also contain a high dose of the amino acid *L-Glutamine*. This amino acid controls cravings and eliminates the desire to eat sweets or sugar. It has been used to control diabetic's glucose levels. Using *L-Glutamine,* there isn't the possibility of "low blood sugar", also known as "hypoglycemia". When you have a METABOLIC PROTEIN™ shake for breakfast, it won't be so easy to "mess up" because your insulin and glucose levels are kept stable. You won't feel hunger or cravings.

The quickest way to boost your metabolism and slim down is to add a dose of COCO-10 PLUS™ to your METABOLIC PROTEIN™ shake. You generally want to prepare it in the morning, with a blender, so that you can combine the two supplements together. COCO-10 PLUS™ doesn't change the flavor of the METABOLIC PROTEIN™ shake.

Take into consideration that the coconut oil in COCO-10 PLUS™ will change to a solid fat if your shake is made cold, by using very cold water or ice cubes. The solution is to blend the METABOLIC PROTEIN™ with the water first and to add the COCO-10 PLUS™ dosage last right before you drink it. This way you don't give the coconut oil enough time to solidify and the shake is creamy and pleasant.

BREAKFAST SHAKE RECIPE

8 ounces water
Dose of COCO-10 PLUS (in tablespoons)
1 o 2 ice cubes (if you like it cold)
2 scoops of METABOLIC PROTEIN

THE POWER OF YOUR METABOLISM

The METABOLIC PROTEIN™ shake mixes well in a blender, but you can also mix it in a closed container, stirring the ingredients until they are well blended. The shake that you drink to replace your breakfast is generally prepared with the following formula:

If you want a thicker or thinner consistency you can increase or decrease the amount of METABOLIC PROTEIN™ that you put in your shake.

For diabetics or people with hypoglycemia (low blood sugar), this shake helps create normal blood glucose levels, which allows both conditions to improve. For other people who use this shake to replace their breakfast, what they notice the most is that their hunger disappears, as well as their desires to eat sweets or refined carbohydrates.

The combination of METABOLIC PROTEIN™ and COCO-10 PLUS™ has the effect of providing you with a superior source of energy to increase your metabolism. The energy and sense of well-being that you feel when you use this shake is notable.

THE STRESS DEFENDER™ SUPPLEMENT

Years of working with thousands of people that had a "slow metabolism" taught us that one of the bigger enemies of the metabolism is STRESS.

At times we live such stressful lives for such long periods of time that we have grown accustomed to the stressful environment and can even consider it "normal" when in fact it is anything but "normal". Economic pressures, family problems, stressful work environments and countless daily bad news impinge on us and cause a stress reaction. The stress reaction forces the body to produce *cortisol*, the so-called "stress hormone".

When there is a high level of *cortisol* running through our body, the thyroid gland is affected, and the metabolism becomes slower, thus we tend to gain fat. When stress has had its toll on us the blood sugar levels have peaks and valleys that make it impossible for us to reduce body fat. When there is too much *cortisol* in our circulation our sleep quality is very poor, and we wake up feeling tired instead of refreshed.

Stress is a killer, but it certainly also makes you fat. To improve on the metabolism, we need to somehow counteract the stress reactions that take our hormonal system out of whack. We need to be free of anxiety and as relaxed as possible to lose weight and slim down.

Through the years, while helping thousands of people to slim down, I have seen the negative effects of stressful situations, like having the wrong marital relationship. Even having to constantly deal with a couple of unruly children can shoot your *cortisol* levels to the sky and make you fat. Stress will effectively sabotage your efforts to slim down.

We tested dozens of different natural substances to help us control the stress reaction of those that wanted to slim down. Some didn't work, others helped only some people and finally we found two natural ingredients that if combined in the correct proportion would produce a calmed state and help the person both slim down and sleep better.

We called it STRESS DEFENDER™. It's a wonderful supplement that in most cases guarantees that the person using the NaturalSlim System will lose the fat they want. We have even had a lot of grateful husbands and wives thanking us because this natural supplement actually helps calm down their stressed-out marriage partner.

This supplement does wonders to help you lose weight, as it controls the body's excessive production of *cortisol*. It shouldn't be used by people who are using the "MAO inhibitor[38]" antidepressant, as the natural L-Tyrosine amino acid that it contains doesn't mix well with this type of antidepressant drug.

---

[38] MAO inhibitor antidepressant – a type of antidepressant drug that is also used for Parkinson's disease. The most common brands are: Marplan, Nardil, Parnate and Eldepryl.

METABOLIC VITAMINS

A s discussed in the section called THE POTENCY OF YOUR VITAMINS IS IMPORTANT, your body will not recover from a "slow metabolism" if you don't give it what it needs to increase the metabolism.

We have seen this at least a thousand times: someone wants to slim down, but they do not want to spend money on a high potency vitamin and mineral formula. So, they run to their nearest Target, Sam's or Costco store and purchase some cheap vitamin formula. Some weeks later the person is disillusioned with the results of their weight loss efforts. At this point the person is feeling gloomy and can't realize that in the subject of the metabolism, you can't cut corners. You need to use a HIGH POTENCY vitamin formula to boost your metabolism or you will fail.

The body is an incredible organism. It's an entity that does its best to survive despite all the damage that we constantly throw its way. Yet, it is an organism that has some basic needs that, if unfulfilled, will eventually hamper its proper functioning. Cars run on gasoline, oil and water. Bodies are a little more complicated in design than a car and need some 30 or more different vitamins and minerals to survive. Some of the body needs are in extremely small quantities like micrograms. A gram weights as much as a paper clip and a microgram is a gram divided in 1,000,000 parts. Yet, if for example, the body needs a very small amount of a mineral like *selenium* and it doesn't get it, then the thyroid gland will be affected, and your metabolism will drop like a rock.

If you can't find a high-potency vitamin and mineral formula in your area, we recommend our METABOLIC VITAMINS. This is a vitamin and mineral formula with a proven track record. People who use them can feel the difference, as it shows itself in their slimmer bodies and an obvious high-energy feeling.

These vitamins are really potent. Thus, they can never be taken on an empty stomach. They go well with your morning METABOLIC PROTEIN™ whey protein shake or with your lunch.

CANDISEPTIC™ KIT:
YEAST CLEANSING PROGRAM

There are a number of people who have not been successful in losing weight mainly due to the fact that their bodies are seriously infected with *candida yeast*. They suffer from irritated, itchy skin (especially at night), sinusitis, migraines, indigestion, flatulence and allergies, along with 20 other symptoms of what doctors refer to as candidiasis, or *yeast infections.* The *candida* yeast produces 78 different toxins inside your body throughout its fermentation process. This creates an environment that is high in acidic substances, which reduces the amount of oxygen in your body and creates a "slow metabolism". People that have a lot of yeast in their bodies typically fail at all of the diets that they go on as a direct result of the excessive amount of yeast that they have in their bodies.

Interestingly enough, no part of the population is more infected with yeast than diabetics. Diabetics, by definition, have high levels of glucose (blood sugar). Since yeast loves to feed on sugar, a diabetics' body is the ideal environment for yeast to grow and it reproduces very quickly. No other part of the population has more yeast in their bodies than people with diabetes. The excess glucose in diabetic's bodies creates a "paradise" for yeast because they find themselves surrounded by an abundant supply of glucose that helps them reproduce.

We've found that when you reduce the amount of yeast in your body, your metabolism speeds up and you slim down much faster with more permanent results. In other words, it is much less likely that you will end up gaining back all of the weight that you lost.

We've created the CANDISEPTIC™ KIT, which is a yeast cleansing system made up of 3 natural supplements:

CANDIDA CLEANSE™ - contains natural fungicidal ingredients that attack the yeast and destroy their ability to reproduce.

GOOD FLORA™ - although it is important to reduce the amount of yeast in your intestinal tract, it is equally important to increase and strengthen the "good bacteria" that make up the intestinal flora. You can't control the yeast in your intestine if you aren't making an effort to keep the "good bacteria" in your intestine strong. The healthy intestinal flora, which is made up of what is called "good bacteria", produces "acidophilin". Acidophilin destroys yeast and protects your intestine from new infections of yeast.

IMMUNE SUPPORT™ - While you are getting rid of the yeast in your body, it unfortunately also creates a toxic environment within your body. This happens because the yeast is dying, decomposing, and then turning into toxins. When there is a strong yeast infection, as in the case of diabetics, the cleansing can be quite unpleasant. As a result, we've created the IMMUNE SUPPORT supplement, which helps improve your body's immune system while promoting the elimination of the toxins through your liver.

Cleansing the yeast from your body can be an uncomfortable experience for you, but with the help of the CANDISEPTIC KIT, it is possible.

FEMME BALANCE™ FOR WOMEN

I n order to help women with their hormones, we've come up with a natural progesterone cream called FEMME BALANCE.

This cream contains natural progesterone and, in some cases, can be considered a "miracle" for women. As explained in this book, the female hormone *estrogen* causes weight gain. This is why women gain weight when they have taken oral contraceptives or hormone replacement medications like Premarin and Prempro. Both oral contraceptives and hormone replacements taken by women going through menopause are made with *estrogen* as the base ingredient.

We already know that *estrogen* can cause or speed up the growth of breast cancer. This is why doctors recommend that women eliminate all sources of estrogen when they discover that they have breast cancer.

Many women suffer from what is called an "estrogen predominance", which Dr. John Lee explains in his book "What your Doctor May Not Tell You About Menopause". In my experience, women who have excess abdominal fat and have a strong tendency to accumulate fat in their hips and thighs are the women who benefit greatly from using the natural *progesterone* cream. Using natural *progesterone* helps women get rid of abdominal fat. This doesn't mean that women have to apply the *progesterone* cream on their abdominal area, since the *progesterone* works with the entire body to fight the negative effects of the estrogen predominance.

When used correctly, the progesterone cream FEMME BALANCE™ can even help women who suffer from hot flashes that they experience when entering menopause. When using it for this purpose, the cream is applied inter-vaginally (inside the vagina) and can effectively control hot flashes.

Natural progesterone has other benefits for women that are just as valuable as those abovementioned. For example, natural *progesterone* helps keep your skin hydrated and restores your skin back to a more youthful appearance. *Progesterone* is like an anti-aging hormone.

Progesterone also has a calming and anti-depressing effect on women. The excess *estrogen* that is produced when a woman has "estrogen predominance" has a stimulating effect and can influence a woman's quality of sleep. Unlike *estrogen*, progesterone helps women sleep more soundly and deeply.

According to Dr. John Lee, when a woman uses *progesterone*, she is preventing the possibility of getting breast cancer. Using progesterone also prevents "estrogen predominance" and therefore reduces the risk of women getting breast cancer.

Finally, *progesterone* naturally boosts the libido (desire to have sex) for women and has been used as a treatment for cases of sexual frigidity. Many men have discovered that *progesterone* has this effect on their wives and make sure that they are using the *progesterone* cream regularly.

TESTOSTERIN™ FOR MEN

Hormones control all of the organs, glands, tissues, muscles, nerves, and bones in your body. Hormones are very powerful substances that can give orders to cells and can therefore modify the structure of your body.

Many of us have heard of athletes who have taken hormones to build more physical strength and endurance. Numerous well-known athletes have been tempted to take steroids (hormones that build muscle). The temptation is great because when a person takes steroids their muscles strengthen and grow, while their enhanced athletic performance gives them an unrivaled competitive advantage. Although it is an illegal and immoral way to compete against other athletes, the temptation is great because every athlete wants to be the best in their sport.

In the scope of natural supplements, there are certain substances that help improve women's hormonal systems and others that help men's hormonal systems.

Women who have the desire to slim down use the natural progesterone cream to reduce the effects of estrogen, which is a feminine hormone that causes weight gain. However, up until now we haven't had anything to help the male hormonal system, and therefore couldn't help those men who wanted to slim down.

We researched and discovered that men could boost their hormonal system if they could manage to naturally increase their production of the masculine hormone *testosterone*. Scientific studies show that after 30 years of age, men gradually start losing the means to produce *testosterone*. For example, it is estimated that by the age of 50, men produce approximately 50% of the amount of *testosterone* that they produced when they were younger. At 60, it lowers to 40%, and at 70 years of age the amount of *testosterone* can be as low as 20% of what they originally produced.

We know that *testosterone* is what creates strong muscles and contributes to a more defined body. This is why as men age they become less muscular and more flaccid, gaining more fat in their bodies. *Testosterone* is a hormone that not only builds big, strong muscles, but it also contributes to reducing body fat. Of all of the bodily tissues, muscles consume the most fat. When men do resistance exercises, like lifting weights, they build muscle and increase their overall muscle mass. Their muscles consume body fat and create a lean, more defined body.

If a man can successfully increase his natural *testosterone* production, he will also succeed in substantially increasing his muscle mass and reducing his body fat. When increasing the production of *testosterone,* it is possible that a man will not be able to lose weight because the new muscles weigh 2.5 times more than fat; however, his body will be slenderer, and he'll have a surplus of energy.

Another benefit from increasing your natural *testosterone* production is that it can have a very positive effect on your sexual health and function. *Testosterone* is the hormone that keeps your sexual interest alive toward your partner, in addition to contributing to the frequency and healthful enjoyment of sexual activity. There are also studies that have shown that men with higher levels of *testosterone* have fewer cardiovascular incidents.

We've created a product called TESTOSTERIN™ in order to help those men who are experiencing problems with their hormones. This product contains a natural extract called TESTOFEN, which in clinical studies has proven to increase *testosterone* production up to 98%. TESTOSTERIN™ contains various ingredients that produce a larger output of *testosterone* and other antioxidants that are used to protect the production of nitric oxide in your body. Nitric oxide is the molecule that allows men to have satisfactory erections and was the discovery that provoked the creation of the medication VIAGRA.

Besides increasing your testosterone levels, TESTOSTERIN™ also boosts your production of nitric oxide. This increase of nitric oxide is not only great for your sexual health and activity, but it also has a relaxing effect on your cardiovascular system. For those individuals who have high blood pressure, it can help regulate the tension in your arteries naturally.

It's also worth mentioning that men that are sexually active have a better attitude toward maintaining their body and their weight. Your emotional state and general attitude toward life are determining factors when it comes to boosting your metabolism and slimming down. Healthy sex between partners promotes attraction and is an excellent outlet to relieve stress. We know that stress produces another hormone called *cortisol* that causes weight gain. Therefore, healthy sexual activity can contribute to both men's and women's health, helping them to slim down without exerting as much effort.

There are several studies that show that *testosterone* levels amongst men who have diabetes are much lower than that of men who don't suffer from diabetes. One of the worst effects of diabetes is that it often causes impotency in men. TESTOSTERIN™ can truly benefit men, especially if they are over 30 years old and suffer from diabetes or high blood pressure.

POTASSIUM KADSORB™

When you do the 2x1 or 3x1 Diet certain specific things happen in your body: the blood glucose levels are reduced, the body produces less insulin (the fattening hormone) and more glucagon (the slimming hormone) and your body starts to break and throw out its excess accumulated fats.

All this is very good because you will feel better and you will also start to become slimmer. But, it isn't that simple. When you start to lose fat, your body also starts to readjust to the new nutrition food mix of the 2x1 or 3x1 Diet. That can, in some cases, make a *potassium* deficiency, shown by a tendency of the body to retain water or swell. In the body, a delicate balance between two minerals maintains the water level, at the cellular level: sodium (salt) and *potassium*. Sodium retains water and *potassium* eliminates water. In the cells the mechanism is called the "sodium-*potassium* pump". Sodium holds on to water, while *potassium* rejects water. Between these two, the body tries to maintain the proper balance.

Sodium is plentiful in most foods, as it is a common preservative. Most prepared foods are high in sodium (salt). *Potassium* is only available in foods like fruits, vegetables or salads.

Most overweight people's bodies are heavily loaded with sodium (salt) and thus they tend to have high blood pressure as sodium retains water and that brings the pressure up in the body. *Potassium* has the opposite effect and acts like a natural diuretic by lowering the blood pressure.

When somebody who is overweight and whose body has accumulated sodium, starts to do the 2x1 or 3x1 Diet, they may notice a swelling or water retention in their body. This is a clear sign of a body that doesn't have enough available *potassium* to counterbalance its stored sodium (salt) reserves.

If you do the 2x1 or 3x1 Diet and notice that your body is retaining water, you need to give your body a *potassium* supplement to help it get rid of the excess sodium (salt). The dosage of *potassium* needed is two 99mg. *potassium* capsules for each 25 pounds of body weight. If your body weighs 200 pounds you would then need 16 daily capsules of *potassium*. One of the clear signs of *potassium* deficiency is having muscle cramps. Muscle cramps are always caused by *potassium* deficiencies.

In my opinion and based on my experience with the thousands of people we have helped to lose weight, it is not dangerous to consume 16 to 20 capsules of potassium per day to compensate for the amount of salt (sodium) intake from foods in your diet. For example, 20 daily capsules, which is what a person that weighs 250 lbs. would take, adds up to 1980 milligrams (20 x 99mg) in total. In comparison, if you ate four bananas a day, you would be consuming a total of 1900 milligrams of potassium, as each contains about 450mg. It is hard to conceive that four bananas a day could put you at risk of a potassium overdose. Thus, we can conclude the same for 20 capsules of potassium, which is what you would consume if your body were at that weight.

In fact, if bananas didn't have such a high carbohydrate count due to the large amount of fructose, I would advise you to eat four per day instead. Unfortunately, however, you will not slim down consuming that many carbohydrates per day. This is why we created KADSORB, a supplement that contains a very absorbable form of potassium that will allow you to counter the sodium intake from your diet and avoid water retention in the body.

A great number of people have reported that, with the help of KADSORB and MAGICMAG, they have been able to reduce high blood pressure and even stabilize arrhythmia (irregular heart beat). The ideal would be to consume a good amount of vegetables and salads each day so as to consume the necessary amount of potassium through your diet. But, however it is consumed, when it comes to improving your metabolism, your body will need the help of potassium to balance out the levels of sodium from your diet. Potassium is important.

"MIRACLE" MAGNESIUM, THE MAGICMAG ® SUPPLEMENT

With her book, *"The Magnesium Factor"*, Dr. Mildred Seelig is definitely the best source of knowledge about the damages that are caused to your health and metabolism due to magnesium deficiencies, and the possible benefits of supplementing your diet with this important mineral. In her book, she explains the close relationship between magnesium deficiencies and high blood pressure, cardiovascular illnesses, diabetes, and other chronic illnesses. The book is full of scientific references and common sense.

I've been working with obesity and metabolism related issues for over 20 years and many things have surprised me, but what has surprised me the most has been the benefits that magnesium can have on some people's health and metabolism.

Many years ago, we discovered in NaturalSlim that there wasn't a more practical solution to constipation than taking magnesium capsules. Constipation is definitely one of the main obstacles that a person can have when trying to slim down. When you are constipated, your body's internal state becomes excessively acidic and toxic, which makes it hard for you to slim down. We've discovered that magnesium capsules help people regulate their bowel movements without causing intestinal irritation and the discomfort that some commonly used natural supplements like "Cáscara Sagrada" can cause.

However, magnesium capsules have one downside: they aren't absorbed very well. Although they are very effective for resolving issues with constipation in nearly 100% of cases, their limitation is that they don't provide enough absorbable magnesium to be able to treat or improve a magnesium deficiency in all of the cells in the body. So, the capsules work great for the intestinal system and for

335

constipation, but they don't provide enough absorption to supplement magnesium to the rest of the body so that it can counteract the magnesium deficiencies that affect people with high blood pressure, cardiovascular problems, muscle pain, diabetes, insomnia, or excessive stress.

According to Dr. Mildred Seelig and what we've been able to prove in those who are overweight or diabetic, magnesium deficiencies can cause the following symptoms:

> Anxiety or nervousness
> Back pain
> Constipation
> Difficulty sleeping; insomnia
> Excessive muscle tension
> Fatigue or weakness
> Headaches; migraines
> High blood pressure
> Irregular heart beat (arrhythmia)
> Low energy
> Low stress tolerance or irritability
> Muscular spasms and cramps
> Premenstrual syndrome (PMS)
> Slow metabolism; difficulty slimming down
> Uncontrollable glucose levels (diabetics)
> Weak bones; Osteoporosis

Magnesium is an essential mineral that you can get through your diet, mainly by eating vegetables and salads. In fact, the color green is the dominating color in plants and in nature, which is caused by the mineral magnesium. Note that the color green is a characteristic of vegetation and is produced by *chlorophyll*[39], which is the green substance that allows plants to capture and use solar

---

[39] Chlorophyll: a pigment (gives color) found in plants and algae. Plants use it to produce the energy that is extracted from solar light. The name comes from the Greek word "cloros", which means "green".

energy to sustain themselves. *Chlorophyll* is green due to its high magnesium content, since magnesium only reflects the green from solar light. This is similar to how iron found in the blood only reflects the color red, which makes blood appear that color.

It's estimated that more than 80% of the population is deficient in magnesium, even though medical professionals have put more emphasis on recommending we supplement our diets with calcium. Calcium is just as important as magnesium for the human body. These two minerals have opposite effects and are both vital for the body. However, what Dr. Seelig explains is that research and clinical studies show that magnesium deficiencies are much more prevalent than calcium deficiencies in our population.

You should know that the absorption of calcium is impossible if you are deficient in magnesium. There are people who are taking high doses of calcium because their doctor recommended that they take calcium supplements for osteoporosis when in reality their bodies can't absorb the calcium due to a magnesium deficiency that is preventing the absorption. The calcium that is ingested and isn't absorbed starts to build up in the tissues, which causes stiffness that can cause an increase in blood pressure due to its calcifying[40] effect in the walls of the arteries. Without magnesium, your body can't absorb calcium.

Magnesium deficiencies are caused by various factors: not eating enough vegetables and salads, emotionally stressful situations, medications (diuretics, antibiotics, contraceptives, insulin, and cortisone, etc.), rigorous exercise, diabetes, digestive problems, or excess calcium in your diet. Many doctors have seen that many of the children who are diagnosed with "Attention Deficit Disorder" or "Hyperactivity" actually have magnesium deficiencies, which results in their nervous system being in a constant state of excitement.

---

[40] Calcify: adds calcium, which hardens cells and takes away flexibility.

In a previous chapter called "We Are All Different", I explained the concept of what an EXCITED nervous system is versus the PASSIVE nervous system, as well as their respective impacts on the human metabolism. Now I would like to explain how magnesium and calcium work together to excite or calm down the nervous system. For example, calcium is the mineral that allows the contraction of the muscles, while magnesium allows the muscles to relax. In a sense, calcium and magnesium actually represent both sides of the same coin.

Those individuals, who have an EXCITED nervous system, or what psychologists call a "Type A" personality, need more magnesium than people who have a PASSIVE system. In fact, people who have PASSIVE nervous systems generally need to increase their consumption of calcium (exciting). Magnesium calms and relaxes while calcium excites and energizes. So, to help fix a serious state of excitement, insomnia, or muscle contractions (muscle spasms), you need to add more magnesium to your diet.

Whenever you undergo stressful situations, the calcium flow to the interior of your cells is increased and the amount of magnesium decreases. There is generally at least 10,000 times more magnesium than calcium in your cells. However, when you are under a lot of stress, the magnesium decreases, and the calcium dominates, which excites the nervous system and contracts your muscular and cardiovascular systems. This increases muscular and vascular (the arteries) tension while raising your blood pressure. This is why bad news or going through a tough time can increase your blood pressure.

Note that the most prominent modern drugs that exist to try to control high blood pressure are called "calcium channel blockers". By blocking the excess calcium that builds up in the walls of the cardiovascular system, these medications have a relaxing affect that lowers your blood pressure. Magnesium is naturally the most efficient "calcium blocker" that the human body has. This is why in many instances you can lower your blood pressure by supplementing your diet with enough magnesium; especially if you take a potassium supplement (potassium is not recommended for people with kidney problems without the supervision of a doctor). Magnesium and potassium work together to activate the so-called "sodium/potassium pump" in the cells, which makes your body urinate the excess sodium (salt) that increases your blood pressure. Generally, your blood pressure decreases significantly if you do this along with drinking an adequate amount of water to hydrate your body to help get rid of the excess sodium (salt) that keeps your blood pressure high. Please, do not try to control your blood pressure or stop taking your blood pressure medication without consulting your doctor. The important point here is that magnesium can help your metabolism and your health, especially when accompanied with a healthy lifestyle.

Diabetics and people who are hypoglycemic (drop in blood sugar) are much more deficient in magnesium than the rest of the population. This is thought to be due to the fact that the human body cannot create the hormone *insulin* without magnesium since magnesium is an essential part of the insulin molecule. People who suffer from depression are also much more deficient in magnesium. Magnesium is essential to over 300 enzymes that the human body needs to function adequately. Many elderly individuals suffer from this deficiency, which is reflected by constipation, muscle pain, weak bones, and difficulty sleeping or relaxing. It has also been found that the human body can't absorb calcium in the bones without the help of magnesium. Many adults suffer from osteoporosis (porous and fragile bones) simply because their body can't absorb calcium as a result of a magnesium deficiency that seems to be an epidemic. Others have found that their arrhythmia (irregular heart beat) improves or goes away when they supplement their diet with magnesium. Magnesium is a mineral that protects the heart and studies show that people who have had heart attacks benefit from taking magnesium supplements. Overall, magnesium can provide many benefits to your health and your metabolism.

I spent a long time looking for a form of magnesium that would be absorbable enough to solve a deficiency that had built up over many years. I finally found the formula that we call MAGICMAG® or "magic magnesium". This magnesium powder is easily absorbed and has a great flavor and is important when you want to supplement your diet with magnesium for a long time, enough to resolve a deficiency. It can be ingested as a tea because it only requires a cup of hot water and it dissolves easily. MAGICMAG® contains *magnesium citrate*, the most absorbable form of magnesium, which has been "ionized" (molecularly activated) so that your cells allow it to be absorbed.

The dose will vary for each person depending on their needs and depending on the individuals' health condition and level of deficiency. You'll start with a small dose of half a teaspoon daily and gradually increase the amount to 3 teaspoons or more a day as needed. It's important to increase the dose gradually to give your body a chance to absorb the magnesium within the cells, which is where it is needed. When you take too much magnesium it causes diarrhea because of its relaxing effect on your intestines. The idea is that each person tries out the different dosages until they find which one is right for their body, which is always the most that can be taken without getting diarrhea. You may be surprised to find that your magnesium deficiency is so severe that you'll take high doses of magnesium for several days before your body gives the signal that you've went over the correct dosage, causing a mild diarrhea.

Magnesium is referred to as "the anti-stress mineral". Certainly, many of us live surrounded by excess stress caused in part by the storm of bad news the media communicates to us on a daily basis. Take your magnesium, take a deep breath, and relax just for a moment and you'll find that your health problems, your diabetes, and your "slow metabolism" can be more easily controlled.

THE CONSTIPEND™ SUPPLEMENT

One of the obstacles, and a factor that causes a "slow metabolism", is having a congested intestine that causes a very slow intestinal movement or what is called "constipation". The least acceptable is to have vowel movement at least once a day. The ideal would be 2 to 3 times per day. When this does not happen, the walls of the intestine begin to line with a sticky and tarry film that makes the absorption of nutrients very difficult. Especially if the person is not used to drinking enough water on a daily basis, the fecal matter compacts against the intestinal walls and that congestion not only prevents the absorption of nutrients, but also creates an extremely acidic state inside the body that results in a slow metabolism.

I'm sorry to say, but that "belly" or abdominal fat that refuses to go away, even when someone exercises their stomach muscles, in many cases is nothing more than the reflection of a congested intestine. Autopsies have shown that fecal matter can expand an intestine's diameter by 2 or 3 times its normal size. An intestine, whose diameter has expanded by 2 or 3 times its normal size due to the accumulation of residue throughout the years, creates in turn a very noticeable and expanded abdomen and of course, it cannot be resolved by exercise because it is not a problem of excess fat, but rather an excess of intestinal reside. Medical doctors who practice autopsies aren't surprised to find grains like corn or other hard-to-digest foods eaten years before in the residue of the intestinal walls.

When the body is excessively toxic due to the accumulation of fecal matter in the walls of the intestines the metabolism is reduced, and the person will not lose weight. In these cases, many problems may arise such as hemorrhoids, or skin allergies, simply because the body is excessively toxic with a congested-up intestine.

The principal cause of cellulite or "orange-peel skin" on the gluts or hips that worries women so much and creates a millionaire market for creams, liposuctions, and a multitude of other remedies, is constipation and the accumulation of fecal matter impacted against the walls of the intestinal tract. The intestines become "a backed-up plumbing system" that accumulates toxins and in addition creates a toxic environment that caters to bacteria, yeast and parasites.

This subject regarding constipation can be an uncomfortable one, but it is necessary that it be understood for the sake of truth. You cannot resolve a problem that you yourself do not even know you have.

Now, women suffer from problems with the thyroid more than men. According to statistics there are 8 women for every 1 man suffering from a thyroid deficiency. This is the reason that constipation affects women more than men. I do not recommend the routine use of laxatives because they work while irritating the delicate intestinal tissue, such as it happens with supplements containing "cáscara sagrada". Very differently from how a laxative works, CONSTIPEND™ is a product formulated to assist with regular intestinal movement, decongest the intestines, clean the intestines of yeast, bacteria and parasites while at the same time helping to regenerate the intestinal tissue.

CONSTIPEND™ works on a basis of decongesting, cleaning and helping to regenerate tissue without causing irritation. When used it in conjunction with the MagicMag® supplement even the most severe cases of constipation can be solved. The deficiency of magnesium that plagues the majority of the population is one of the principal reasons for the problem of constipation.

In order to have a good metabolism you must avoid the accumulation of toxins in the intestines by achieving an adequate bowel movement and for this purpose CONSTIPEND™ can be of great help.

Helpzymes™

When it comes to improving your metabolism, it is important to know that what nourishes your body is not just what you eat, but what your body can digest and absorb. In order for a certain type of food (such as protein, carbohydrates, or fat) and its nutrients (vitamins and minerals) to serve as fuel for the metabolism, they must first be absorbed. There are numerous people with a "slow metabolism" whose principal problem is poor digestion and, in this case, not even the best foods or nutrients will be of any benefit.

It is common amongst those who are overweight, obese or diabetic, to experience digestive problems such as acid reflux, intestinal gases, constipation, stomach acid, and even body odor due to the foods that end up rotting inside the body as a result of poor digestion. The pharmaceutical industry promotes all kinds of "antacid" medication because poor digestion is a very common problem that worsens with age. Amongst the elderly, the problem can become chronic and many do not respond to good nutrition simply because their digestive system does not do what it is supposed to.

To make matters worse, it has been discovered that with age, many of us begin to suffer from an inefficient production of hydrochloric acid in the stomach. This acid, which is vital to digestion, is what allows food to be absorbed by the cells in the body. In combination with digestive enzymes, the metabolism will then be able to actually use these nutrients.

Those who have experienced digestive problems such as stomach acid can probably remember a time when they could eat almost anything and not suffer from bad digestion or acidity. But, with many years of abuse to the digestive system, such as by consuming sugar, candy, and sodas, combined with years of poor hydration can take a toll on the digestive system until it becomes inefficient.

Digestion is a VITAL process that can make the difference between good health and a body full of energy, or an ill and weak body with a "slow metabolism", which becomes lethargic and obese. If we were to compare a body to a car we would say that the food, we eat is the fuel or gasoline for the body and that digestion is equivalent to what a carburetor does in a car's motor; it makes fuel available to the motor so that it can be used as energy. Even if you fill up your gas tank with the best available gas in the world, your car will not produce good energy if the carburetor does not do its job of providing gasoline in a useable form. It's the same situation when it comes to digestion. If your digestion is not working well, not even the 2x1 Diet or 3x1 Diet will save you. To have a strong metabolism you need to have strong digestion.

Also, the hydrochloric acid produced by your stomach prevents bacteria and parasites hidden in the food you eat from surviving inside of your body. In other words, this stomach acid is an integral part of your immune system. For this reason, people who suffer from poor digestion have more bacterial infections and parasites, which in turn reduces the metabolism and worsen conditions such as diabetes.

We have worked with many people throughout the years with digestive problems, which led to a continued "slow metabolism" and slow recuperation from any illnesses they had. I began to look into what was happening with these people who were not improving as fast as others and discovered that many of them were suffering from a compromised digestive system. I began to search for ways of helping them and discovered that it would be to their advantage to supplement their diet with digestive enzymes and hydrochloric acid.

I worked with experts in the field of digestive enzymes and was able to develop a supplement to help these people recuperate their digestion. This supplement contains various proteolyctic (helps digest proteins) digestive enzymes as well as other enzymes to help efficiently digest carbohydrates, oils and fats. This digestive enzyme and hydrochloric supplement is called HELPZYMES™. For those with acid reflux, fatigue after a meal (due to poor digestion), stomach acid, or body odor, HELPZYMES can be of much benefit.

When I was formulating HELPZYMES™ I realized that the supplement industry is full of unethical products, in the sense that many manufactures pretended to offer digestive enzymes without the ability to prove the ACTIVITY of such enzymes. For example, some attempted to sell digestive enzymes "by weight", which is illogical as it is not the enzyme's weight or quantity that helps create good digestion but its PROVEN ACTIVITY to digest proteins, carbohydrates or fats. After a lot of searching, I found reliable manufacturers that could provide us with a laboratory analysis that certified the level of digestive ACTIVITY in the enzymes. Money motivation exists even in the field of "natural products", which of course, results in a market full of products that promise help it can't deliver.

HELPZYMES™ were especially formulated to help people with a "slow metabolism", which is why it has a large number of enzymes, such as "pancreatine", to help digest proteins that will activate your metabolism. It is also reinforced with "lipase", an enzyme that breaks up fats to help a person slim down and contribute in the disposal of triglycerides or fats that accumulate in the walls of the arteries.

The results achieved with HELPZYMES™ are very noticeable. A person, who once suffered from digestive problems or stomach acid, will begin to see how he or she can now eat less food and yet feel less hungry as a result of improved digestion and overall absorption of nutrients. HELPZYMES™ are not necessarily always needed for the entirety of your life, as the digestive system's ability to recuperate can improve as your "life style" changes and when hydration is handled as proposed in this book.

A deficient production of hydrochloric acid is intimately associated with thyroid gland problems. Problems with this gland reduce the production of hydrochloric acid in the stomach, thus creating inefficient digestion that worsens an already "slow metabolism". Thus, we reinforced HELPZYMES™ with a dose of hydrochloric acid because we well know that many of those who suffer from a slow metabolism problem are also suffering from a deficient thyroid gland.

When it comes to improving your metabolism, digestion and absorption are VITAL.

GLOSSARY- DEFINITIONS OF WORDS

Adaptogen (definition): a natural substance that allows the body to counter adverse physical, chemical, or biological stressors by raising resistance toward such stress, thus allowing the organism to "adapt" to the stressful circumstances. Adaptogens are a natural herb product that increases the body's resistance to stresses such as trauma, anxiety and bodily fatigue. Some adaptogens have been shown to help weight loss and even cancer in government sponsored studies that were secretly done in Russia since 1940.

Carbohydrates (definition): carbohydrates are foods like breads, rice, potatoes, yams, starches, and different flours of grains (corn, wheat, barley, etc.), pasta, vegetables, fruits, and sugars. By definition, carbohydrates are sugar molecules like glucose, fructose and lactose among others. The human body uses glucose (blood sugar, carbohydrates) as a source of energy for the cells. They are called "carbohydrates" because they contain the elements carbon and hydrogen, together with oxygen.

Cholesterol (definition): a natural substance that humans and animals produce. Cholesterol is the main construction material of many different hormones like *estrogen* (female hormone) and *testosterone* (male hormone). Nearly all cells in the body contain cholesterol except bone cells. There is a cholesterol called "good cholesterol" (HDL, *high density lipoprotein)* and one called "bad cholesterol" (LDL, *low density lipoprotein).*

Cortisol (definition): This hormone is produced in the adrenal glands, which are found in the area above the kidneys. It is produced in response to stress and its effect includes actions like increased blood glucose levels (that's why it makes us fat), destroying various muscles by turning them into amino acids that the body can use to produce energy (the destruction of the muscles causes flabby skin), lowering the action of the immune system (creating a higher probability of bacterial infections, viruses, fungi, or parasites) and reducing any inflammation in the body. It is called "the stress hormone".

Enzyme (definition): Enzymes are proteins that participate in changes and transformations of other substances. For example, there is an enzyme that transforms and turns cholesterol into the hormone *estrogen*. There are different enzymes that are used to digest fats, proteins and carbohydrates. There are enzymes in the body whose main function is to disable toxic substances that penetrate the body. Some enzymes break the bonds that exist between food atoms and this frees the energy that the food contains. There are enzymes involved in all of the body's processes.

Goitrogens (definition): natural or chemical substances that have been shown to suppress the functions of the thyroid gland. Anything that negatively affects the function of the thyroid gland also lowers the metabolism. Some natural goitrogens are found in soy. One of the substances that lowers the thyroid's production of hormones is the fluoride found in toothpaste.

Hyperthyroidism (definition): a condition in which the thyroid gland produces an excess of the thyroid hormones. This causes weight loss, palpitations, high blood pressure, insomnia, panic attacks, difficulty concentrating and constant tiredness and nervousness, among other things.

Hypoglycemia (definition): the word "hypoglycemia" means, "low blood sugar". The prefix "hypo" means "low" and "glycemia" comes from "glucose". Contrary to diabetics who have too high glucose levels, people with hypoglycemia at times have glucose levels that are too low. Having low glucose levels causes shaking, dizziness, sweating and mental disorientation. It is thought that practically all diabetics were hypoglycemic before becoming diabetics.

Hypothyroidism (definition): a condition in which the thyroid gland doesn't produce enough of the hormones that control the metabolism and body temperature. This condition is characterized by symptoms like depression, hair loss, and coldness in extremities, constipation, dry skin, difficulty slimming down, constant tiredness, digestive problems and continual infections. It is a condition that isn't always detected in laboratory tests and can exist sub- clinically (without being detected by a lab test).

Insulin (definition): a very important hormone that is produced in the pancreas and allows glucose to be transported to the cells to be used as a source of energy for the body. It is the hormone that allows fat to build up in the body when there is an excess of glucose that isn't used by the cells. Diabetics have problems related to this hormone and in some cases have to inject themselves with it if their pancreas has already suffered damage and doesn't produce enough of it.

Metabolism (definition): the sum of all of the processes and chemical changes that your body uses to convert food and nutrients into energy to survive. *Movement* is the word that best defines *metabolism*. The *metabolism* has to do with all of the *movements* in the human body. The origin of the word is from the Greek *"meta"* which means "change" or "movement".

Osteoporosis (definition): condition in which bone loss occurs in the body. This condition mainly affects women that are going through menopause. Pore-like lesions start forming in the bones, which contribute to the bone loss and increase the risk of bone fractures from simple falls or bumps.

Polyunsaturated oils (definition): oils and fats are made up of molecules of carbon, hydrogen, and oxygen atoms. When all of the carbon atoms of oil are joined with hydrogen atoms it is then called a saturated fat (pig fat, coconut oil, etc.). If there are carbon atoms that aren't joined to hydrogen atoms, then the oil is polyunsaturated oil (corn oil, vegetable oil, etc.). The oils that are not saturated (covered) by hydrogen and that have carbon atoms that can be accessed by oxygen atoms react to the oxygen in the environment and can oxidize and decompose. The polyunsaturated oils are those oils that contain a large amount of carbon atoms that are free from hydrogen atoms and therefore can react to the oxygen in the environment and oxidize and decompose if they aren't refrigerated.

Proteins (definition): proteins are foods like meat, cheese and eggs. Proteins are made up of amino acids. Several amino acids together build a protein. Many hormones, like insulin, are proteins. Digestive enzymes are also proteins that are made up of amino acids. The word "protein" originates from the Greek word *"protas"*, which means "of utmost importance".

Root vegetables (definition): foods like tapioca, turnips, potatoes, beets, sweet potatoes, yams and others that grow underground and that are made up of mainly starches. Starches are sugar molecules that very easily turn into glucose.

Starches (definition): Starches are molecules made up of simple sugars, which the body very easily turns into glucose (blood sugar). Rice, yams, potatoes and turnips are all starches.

Triglycerides (definition): triglycerides are fats. All fats and oils are triglycerides. They are called triglycerides because the molecules that make up all fats and oils always contain 3 (tri) extension lines made up of fatty acids hooked to a backbone of glycerin. That's where the word *triglyceride* comes from. What determines if it is olive oil, corn oil, a human blood fat or another type of oil depends on the type of fatty acid that makes up the extension.

Whey protein (definition): various types of proteins are extracted from milk, like casein and whey. Whey has been proven to be the type of protein that speeds up the metabolism the most; therefore, consuming it has a protecting effect, because it powers the body's immune system. There isn't any other protein that is more appropriate to lose weight or improve the metabolism than whey protein.

RECOMMENDED READING
AND INFORMATION RESOURCES

Adaptogens:
The Scientific Validation of Herbal Medicine – Daniel B. Mowrey, Ph. D.

Artic Root (Rhodiola Rosea) The Powerful New Ginseng Alternative – Carl Germano, R.D., C.N.S., L.D.N. and Zakir Ramazanov. Ph. D.

The Rhodiola Revolution – Richard P. Brown, M.D. and Patricia L. Gerbarg, M.D.

Effective Natural Stress and Weight Management Using Rhodiola Rosea and Rhododendron Caucasicum – Dr. Zakir Ramazanov and Dr. María del Mar Bernal Suárez

Candida albicans yeast:
The Yeast Connection Handbook – William G. Crook, M.D.

Candida albicans: The Quiet Epidemic – Stanley Weinberger, C.M.T.

The Yeast Syndrome – John Parks Trowbridge, M.D. and Morton walker, D.P.M.

The Missing Diagnosis – C. Orian Truss, M.D.

Carbohydrate addictions:
The Hidden Addiction and How to Get Free – Janice Keller Phelps, M.D. and Alan E. Nourse, M.D.

Sugar Blues – William Dufty

The Carbohydrate Addict's Diet - Rachael F. Heller and Richard F. Heller

Coconut oil:
The Healing Miracles of Coconut Oil – Bruce Fife, N.D.

Eat Fat Look Thin - Bruce Fife, N.D.

CoQ10:
The Coenzyme Q10 Phenomenon– Stephen T. Sinatra, M.D., F.A.C.C.

Cortisol and stress:
The Stress of Life- Hans Selye, M.D. (Nobel Peace Prize Winner in Physics in 1967)

The Cortisol Connection – Shawn Talbott, Ph. D.

Diabetes:
Dr. Bernstein's Diabetes Solution - Richard K. Bernstein, M.D.

Relationship between different sicknesses and nutrition:
Nutrition and Physical Degeneration – Weston A. Price, D.D.S

Life Without Bread – Christian B. Allan, Ph. D. & Wolfgang Lutz, M.D.

Fats and oils:
Fats that Heal, Fats that Kill – Udo Erasmus

Food intolerances:
False Fat Diet – Elson M. Haas, M.D.

Importance of water:
Your Body's Many Cries for Water – F. Batmanghelidj, M.D.

L-Tyrosine and L-Glutamine Amino acids:
The Healing Nutrients Within – Eric R. Braverman, M.D.

Milk:
Don't Drink Your Milk! – Frank A. Oski, M.D.

Nutrition to slim down:
Protein Power – Michael R. Eades, M.D. and Mary Dam Eades. M.D.

Progesterone hormone:
What Your Doctor May Not Tell You About Menopause – John R. Lee, M.D.

Natural Progesterone – John R. Lee, M.D.

Stagnant metabolism:
Natural Hormonal Enhancement – Rob Faigin

Thyroid problems:
Thyroid Power – Richard L. Shames, M.D. and Karilee Halo Shames, R.N., Ph. D.

The Thyroid Diet – Mary J. Shomon

Wilson's Temperature Syndrome – E. Denis Wilson, M.D.

Solved: The Riddle of Illness – Stephen E. Langer, M.D. and James F. Scheer

Hypo-thyroidism: The Unsuspected Illness – Broda O. Barnes, M.D. and Lawrence Galton

Trampoline:
The Miracles of Rebound Exercise – Albert E. Carter

Rebound Exercise, The Ultimate Exercise for The New Millenium – Albert E. Carter

Vitamins, minerals, and natural herbs:
New Vitamin Bible – Earl Mindell, R.P.H., Ph.D.

Supplement Bible – Earl Mindell, R.P.H., Ph.D.

The Miracle of Magnesium – Carolyn Dean, M.D., N.D.

Encyclopedia of Nutritional Supplements – Michael T. Murray, N.D.

Clear Body, Clear Mind – L. Ron Hubbard

The Real Vitamin & Mineral Book – Shari Lieberman, Ph., CNS, FACN and Nancy Bruning

ADDITIONAL RESOURCES

NaturalSlim USA
www.us.NaturalSlim.com
1200 Starkey Road Suite #205
Largo, Florida 33771
Telephone 1-888-348-7352 (1-888-FIT-RELAX)
e-mail: info@relaxslim.com
To receive intensive, personalized, and professional help if you have already experienced various failures due to a slow metabolism, diabetes, or hypothyroidism. Also, to know more or order special supplements like RELAXSLIM, METABOLIC PROTEIN, COCO-10 PLUS, STRESS DEFENDER, METABOLIC VITAMINS, THYROL and to order progesterone cream, magnesium or potassium supplements so as to boost your metabolism and slim down.

NaturalSlim, Inc.
San Juan, Puerto Rico
Telephone: 1-787-763-2527
www.NaturalSlim.com (site is in Spanish)
To receive intensive, personalized, and professional help if you have already experienced various failures due to a slow metabolism, diabetes, or hypothyroidism.

Carlos Cidre, M.D.
Internal Medicine Specialist – Board Certified
Manatí, Puerto Rico
Telephone 1-787-884-3139
Dr. Cidre is an Internal Medicine Specialist that also treats the subclinical hypothyroidism using Dr. Denis Wilson's system to restore the thyroid function. He also treats other conditions related to obesity, like diabetes and high blood pressure. Dr. Cidre is also a *Certified Metabolism Consultant (CMC)*.

www.MetabolismoTV.com
MetabolismoTV is an Internet TV Channel and interactive video blog where Frank discusses topics about health and metabolism, and the latest discoveries in these areas. These videos can also be watched in our YouTube Channel www.youtube.com/MetabolismoTV and on the MetaTV app for iPhone. (Videos are in Spanish)

Metabolism University   **www.MetabolismUniversity.com**
Metabolism University (UNIMETAB) is the most complete virtual study center that exists on the topics of metabolism and health. UNIMETAB offers courses, from basic to advanced, which are in the investigations and discoveries of the obesity and metabolism specialist, Frank Suárez.

The courses have videos, special educations made by Frank, studies and illustrative photos of each concept, practice exercises, study guide and an official diploma signed by Frank. The courses of UNIMETAB can be done in the mobile equipment, computer and computer, in the time in which each person is more convenient 24/7. The material of the course can be revised or used as a future reference, since it can be accessed permanently for the students of the Metabolism University.

Visit us at www.MetabolismUniversity.com

INDEX

tumor necrosis factor-alpha 130
turkey   34, 43, 171, 214, 218
type F (fattening) food   185
type S (slimming) foods   185, 187, 188
unhealthy body   161
uric acid   282
vaginal flora   116, 121, 122
vegetable juice   213, 214
vegetable oil   34, 97, 98, 350
vegetables 34, 35, 51, 53, 55, 62, 113, 127, 169, 172, 189, 197, 199, 201, 213, 214, 218, 230, 331, 347, 350
vegetarianism   33
vested interests   128
Viagra   71, 329
viruses   116, 291, 348
vitamin B-12   175
vitamins 52, 78, 85, 152, 169, 170, 173, 174, 175, 176, 213, 266, 287, 293, 295, 305, 306, 315, 321, 322
VLDL cholesterol   226
waistline   25, 89, 158, 160, 161, 208
walking92, 141, 144, 145, 213

water   34, 37, 43, 65, 66, 67, 68, 69, 70, 71, 94, 95, 101, 107, 108, 121, 138, 143, 157, 158, 163, 164, 169, 197, 213, 218, 219, 269, 276, 287, 293, 302, 311, 317, 321, 331, 332, 354
water retention   75, 108, 133
weakness   62, 76, 107, 118, 268
wheat   33, 52, 104, 106, 107, 108, 128, 172, 192, 213, 347
whey protein   35, 106, 112, 213, 303, 315, 316, 322, 351
whiskey   123
white meat   171
whole wheat   192
wine   34, 69, 123
withdrawal syndrome   220
www.drugstore.com   83
Xenical®   265
yeast colony   120, 121
yeasts 27, 91, 115, 116, 117, 119, 124, 284, 305, 313
zinc   78, 85, 175, 176, 265
Zolof®   137